P9-DDF-561

LESLEY KINZEL

TWO
WHOLE
CAKES

How to Stop Dieting and
Learn to Love Your Body

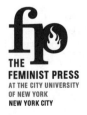

**THE
FEMINIST PRESS**
AT THE CITY UNIVERSITY
OF NEW YORK
NEW YORK CITY

Published in 2012 by the Feminist Press
at the City University of New York
The Graduate Center
365 Fifth Avenue, Suite 5406
New York, NY 10016

feministpress.org

First printing January 2012

Cover design by Herb Thornby, herbthornby.com
Text design by Drew Stevens

Library of Congress Cataloging-in-Publication Data

Kinzel, Lesley, 1977-
Two whole cakes : how to stop dieting and learn to love
your body / Lesley Kinzel.
    p. cm.
ISBN 978-1-55861-793-3
1. Overweight women—Psychology. 2. Body image in
women. 3. Self-esteem in women. I. Title.
RC552.O25K53 2012
616.3980082—dc23

                                                2011040807

In memory of Jill Taylor

I cannot remember a time in my life when I didn't know I was fat. It is an understanding that has pressed down on me with more gravity than anything else ever could. Our culture is steeped in ideologies of aspiration and one of the most inescapable is the pressure to meet narrow standards of beauty and health, standards that are arbitrary and often damaging.

But wait! you object, *don't you know there's an obesity epidemic?* It's impossible not to know. All over the media, fatness is heralded as a major health crisis, a mounting threat to the American way of life. Hell, it's the end of human civilization. Even our children are fat! It is unthinkable. In a contemporary reworking of ancient combat in which the crowd cheers for the lions, fat people are tormented by screaming fitness trainers on national television and people tune in by the millions to watch with unrestrained delight as offensive bodies are elevated from fat sin to starving, dehydrated sainthood. Like modern-day gladiators, these combatants battle fiercely not with an external enemy, but with themselves. This is no longer just an "obesity epidemic" as defined by those who'd seek to pathologize and condemn our bodies. It is a fat rampage. And some fat people are responding in kind. Fat people are finding their voices, standing up, speaking out, and taking back their bodies.

This book is a transmission from that battlefield. It is a product of ten years of discussions, arguments, and revelations taking place in and around body acceptance and social justice movements. It is an analysis of intersectional identities and the complex realities of survival as a self-accepting person in a world that loathes self-acceptance. It is my story. It is also the story of many others who have fought for recognition and respect, and the right to live in their own bodies according to their own desires. It is memoir, conversation, cultural critique, and self-acceptance instruction manual.

According to the dubious measurements of the body mass index (BMI) scale, I am morbidly obese. To put it more succinctly, I am death fat. I am super-duper really-for-real mad fat. I am the kind of fat where doctors are friendly until they get me on a scale, and then after that they get very quiet. *Oh,* I imagine them thinking, *I didn't realize you were that fat.* I am the kind of fat that occasionally outsizes plus-size shops. I am the kind of fat that people reference when they say, "Well, some people are just big, but people who are REALLY fat are just not normal or healthy, and those people SHOULD lose some weight." When they say this sort of thing, they are talking about me.

Furthermore, I adore cooking and refuse to keep anything less than real butter in my house. I eat very little meat but not for moral or ideological reasons; I just dislike preparing it. My diet consists primarily of fresh vegetables and whole grains, and I have a serious weakness for good cheese. I keep a jar of bacon fat in my refrigerator and I occasionally use it to cook big leafy greens, because big leafy greens do best with a bit of bacon fat. I exercise; I have a gym membership and I use it. I take the stairs at work five or six times a day, but only because I am too impatient to wait for the elevator. By the tests and non-BMI numbers doctors use to measure such things, I am healthy.

I have a partner who unconditionally supports my self-acceptance, while struggling with his own. I have a decidedly not-fat family that is mostly supportive of my choices and realities except for the very occasional lapse into the "but I'm just worried about your health" rhetoric.

I have been fat in varying degrees my whole life. Though I've lost and regained many a pound, I've never lost enough weight to feel a glimmer of what it might be like to be thin. I've never lost enough weight to come close to being not fat. Never enough to shop in not-fat stores. Never enough that I wouldn't occasionally hear "fat bitch" hollered at me from a moving car when walking alone, on a city street, or in a parking lot. Never enough that a doctor's ever said I was of a normal weight. Never enough that I didn't, even for a second, feel like I wasn't fat anymore.

Now some folks will read this and think, *oh, how sad.* But there's no sadness here. I am, plainly, morbidly obese. Death fat. I say this without judgment and without disdain. I say it not with an eager ring of reclamation, nor with self-loathing and fear. It just is. I live fully in this real and complicated world.

This is a book about many things, but it is mostly about refusing to be sorry.

There exists a social justice movement focused on criticizing our conventional wisdom about bodies and fat, and on changing our culture to create space where a diversity of bodies is respected and normalized. Different folks call this ideology by different names—fat activism, fat acceptance, fat liberation, fat advocacy. The common ground we all stand upon is the desire for fat bodies—and all bodies, no matter their circumstances—to be seen as worthy of dignity and respect. Fat politics is a movement of criticism and questions, not authority and groupthink. Its purpose ought to be noisy inquiry into what our culture tells us about bodies. Its purpose is not to replace one set of monolithic rules with another. We want fatness to be disentangled from its association with moral decrepitude, and for fat bodies to be understood as valid—not temporary, not disposable, and not loathsome.

Your body is not a tragedy.

This is important. This is something you should know before we go any further. Speak it aloud if it helps. Write it down. Tell someone, "My body is not a tragedy." Whatever else it might be, it is not tragic. Tragedy may yet befall it, or may have already done so, but your body is not the things that happen to it, the things that are forced upon it, or even its failures to perform to certain standards. Your body simply is. The tragedy is the effort required to build a loving relationship—or at least one of tacit acceptance—with your body. In a more perfect world, this connection would take place organically, but any such connection built in our early years is rapidly undone as we learn to criticize and dissociate from our bodies. Then we must spend our remaining years trying to rebuild that relationship.

This world is filled with bodies—in droves, shoulder to shoulder, leaning into and against the crush of daily life—and all of them are different. We're taught that our differences are a weakness, our downfall, and that striving for sameness is the path to happiness and success. No. Humanity is diverse, wonderfully so, and the everlasting battle of fighting our bodies, of fighting ourselves, damages us.

Every day we wake up in our bodies, and we begin to tell our stories. This book collects some of them.

Once upon a time there was a Misguided Young Woman who entered a very large and active fat-positive online space that I was co-moderating. In this space, Misguided was a habitual troublemaker, continuously flouting two of the community's most basic rules: one, don't talk about dieting; and two, don't say mean or critical things about your body or anyone else's body. The team of moderators gave her numerous second chances, far more than she deserved. We did so because the forum had proven its ability to be truly transformative—often the people who are most resistant to the rules at first, later come to appreciate how these guidelines operate to make the space as awesome as it is.

Unfortunately, Misguided could not control herself, and eventually, with heavy hearts, my co-moderators and I decided to ban her permanently, to the relief and cheers of thousands of other community members.

About a year later, I was reading a comment thread elsewhere online when I ran across an exchange between Misguided, whom I had nearly forgotten about, and a few other people. As it happened, Misguided was telling the story of being banned from our online community. She seemed to be under the impression that she was banned for daring to question the right of fat people to eat cake.

"These people eat, like, a whole cake in one sitting. That's not right!" wrote Misguided.

Of course, this was silly. The other commenters interacting with Misguided were mostly dismissive, saying, "What business is it of mine what someone eats? I don't really care."

Exasperated, Misguided responded, with her characteristic hyperbole, "SO YOU THINK IT'S TOTALLY

OKAY FOR FAT PEOPLE TO EAT TWO WHOLE CAKES EVERY DAY?"

There was something about the absurdity of this question that captured my imagination. Thus the concept of "two whole cakes" was born. Originally, it was an in-joke between me and my friends, and then it became a popular shout-out in fat communities online. Shortly thereafter #twowholecakes first appeared as a hashtag on Twitter, and suddenly I started seeing it everywhere, bandied back and forth between people I didn't know on various online forums, even getting a mention during an "obesity epidemic" debate on *Nightline*.

So what does it mean?

The phrase "two whole cakes" is appealing because it is ridiculous. It evokes the kind of insatiable appetite and gratuitous pleasure seeking that our culture so erroneously assigns to fat people. It suggests a total loss of self-control, the danger that—as Marianne Kirby has put it—fat people will "eat the whole world."

It is also very funny. It's useful to zero in on negative stereotypes and show how preposterous they are. That's my kind of activism: to create ideas that spread like airborne viruses, that multitudes can grab onto and carry around like a secret or an answer to a question that few ever dare to ask.

To me, two whole cakes represents the absurd hyperbole associated with weight and body size. It acknowledges that there are folks out there who sincerely believe that all fatasses everywhere do things like sit down and eat two whole cakes on a regular basis, whence their fatness is maintained or improved upon. The over-the-topness of not one, but *two* whole cakes highlights the ridiculousness of beating myself up for making personal choices that do no real damage other than to offend conventional wisdom. Did you eat something yesterday that you're judging yourself harshly for? Stop. Did you say or think something critical about someone else's eating habits or their body? Think about why you did that and how you feel when someone does it to you. Did someone say something damaging to you that's lingering in the back of your mind? Acknowledge why it hurt, and move on.

Two whole cakes is about giving up and letting go of all the self-hating garbage we carry around inside our heads, and finding acceptance and contentment as we are now. *Even if we've eaten two whole cakes.*

I gave a talk about two whole cakes in 2010, and afterward an acquaintance emailed me to ask, "But what if someone actually wanted to eat two whole cakes? Publicly? What happens when the cartoonish caricature is made real?" It is not my place to judge others for making autonomous decisions about what they do with their bodies. Nor is it yours. Because ultimately, you or I could eat two whole cakes and probably the worst thing that would come of it is that we'd feel terribly sick afterward. But our lives wouldn't end. We wouldn't be bad people. We wouldn't have anything to apologize for. It is no one's business but our own.

I don't advocate eating two whole cakes on a regular basis, but the phrase, to me, captures something of the wild freedom and relief I felt when I was first discovering fat acceptance. It reminds me of the way those simple concepts—eating what I wanted, when I was hungry, without feeling guilty, and stopping when I was done; not hating myself or my body; building a critical resistance to the cultural messages around me—have created a revolution within me. I could eat two whole cakes if I wanted to! I don't want to, but I could, if I did. Two whole cakes is about laughing at the stereotypes and assumptions that hurt us and thereby lessening their power to do so. Pass it on. Tell your friends. Reinvent it for your own purposes. Two whole cakes is a force that can't be denied.

At some point in the unfolding of human history, it was decided that fat girls are not supposed to wear dresses. Or colors other than black. Or horizontal stripes. Or ruffles, or florals, or knee socks, or wide belts. No heels, no flats, no skinny jeans, no palazzo pants. Nothing too tight and nothing too big. Nothing too bright. Nothing too trendy.

There are a great many rules for fat-lady dressing. These rules—shared in deferential whispers, with religious fervor, and agreed upon as irrefutable truths—make the clothing available to fat people lacking in imagination and variety. These rules make dressing a fat body often a Brobdingnagian challenge, which occasionally involves the identification of one's body shape with a piece of produce (are you an apple? a pear? I am a butternut squash) and the constant battle of refusing to live in wrap dresses *even though everyone knows wrap dresses are incredibly flattering*.

"Flattering" and "unflattering" are so overused and underdefined that they've come to stand as code for opinions that might be offensive or hurtful if stated in clearer terms. One might argue that a "flattering" ensemble is one that suits an individual in a way that makes him or her feel comfortable, confident, and generally fabulous, and underscores and shares his or her existing, internal awesomeness with the outside world. It's possible that "flattering" evokes this idea, some of the time. But just as often it translates to "that makes you look thinner," or more proportional, or otherwise makes your body look in a way that it does not ordinarily look. Further, when we say something is unflattering, we're often trying to deliver bad news in a polite way, by deflecting blame from the body to the garment, in spite of the fact that most of us are going to secretly blame the body anyway. Women in particular are prone to directing their anger at themselves rather than at the pair of jeans that fails to fit both their hips and waist at the same time, as though the jeans' expectations must necessarily prevail over the actual dimensions of the body you've had for your entire life. If the jeans don't fit, it must be *your* fault. You should change to fit them, because the jeans are in charge here. If you refuse—silly, stubborn person that you are—then you are relegating yourself to fashion struggles in perpetuity.

Fashion is communication. If you cannot fit fashion, then you are left out of the conversation. Imagine you're at a dinner party with ten amazing people; they are having fascinating discussions on topics that interest you, but when you try to join in, no one listens. They talk over you. They don't even notice you're there. This is something of what it's like to be a fashionably minded fat woman.

In the interconnected worlds of fashion media and fashion design, fat women are typically presumed to be not merely incapable of style, but a direct assault on everything fashion stands for. Karl Lagerfeld, a member of fashion's old guard who currently heads up the timeless entity that is Chanel, has declared, with a characteristic lack of subtlety, "No one wants to look at fat women." High fashion and the arbiters of style have a built-in fat ceiling beyond which no body past a particular size (an eight? a ten? a—*gasp*—twelve?) may pass. Fat people lack any kind of comparable access to stylish and well-fitting clothes, not simply because those clothes are expensive—and they are—but because they don't exist. Certainly, there are a handful of committed plus-size designers who make quality apparel out there, but the plus options are a tiny fraction of what is available to non-plus people. And while some heinously overpriced knitwear for up-to-a-size-twenty-four fat folks can be found at a premium in the darkest, dustiest basement corner of the occasional high-end department store (or, failing that, on the store's website), the selection even among the $400 polyester jersey dresses is—to put it delicately—unimpressive. In recent years, Beth Ditto, the unapologetically fat and queer lead singer of the dance-punk band Gossip, has been unexpectedly embraced by the fashion world. Even Karl Lagerfeld had her band play at an event (though we can suppose he avoided looking directly at the stage the whole time). As a result, Ditto has come to serve as a rare icon of fat style; designers specially produce clothing for her, either for the stage, or for a feature in a magazine. But I think Ditto is only accepted as an iconoclast because she is seen as an aberration. Her inclusion in the conversation does not signal the coming around of high fashion to embrace fat women as a whole; in fact, I would argue that it further ensures that won't happen, since including fats aplenty would erase the novelty that Ditto's fatness currently supplies. I suppose this is just as well because if I try to put myself, accustomed to waging straight-up war in an attempt to cultivate a personal style out of the lemons mainstream plus-size clothing manufacturers offer me, in Ditto's position, in which I might suddenly have Chanel call and offer to make me a dress, I cannot imagine my response. Would years of rage spill out of me in a stream of vile profanity? Would I humbly blubber my thanks and send my measurements right over? I can't even imagine.

The truth is, it's practically impossible, even for

fat people of means, to ever truly meet the standards set by the magazines and designers who tell us what is stylish. And it's not only because fat people are presumed inherently sloppy or uninterested in clothing. It's because in addition to having few options for clothing—they are simply fat. Within these circles, fat itself is unfashionable, and no garment, no matter how dramatic or expensive, can overcome that fact.

Once a reader asked me how she might deal with her reluctance to wear dresses and heels, because, as a fat person, doing so made her feel like "an elephant in drag."

I really enjoyed this analogy.

The clash between fat and femininity is a common issue for many fat people who'd like to dress in more feminine ensembles. Culturally speaking, fatness is perceived as anti-feminine. Interestingly, it is also antimasculine in men, so it seems that whatever your intended gender presentation may be, fatness is going to fuck with it. Though male-identified people are hardly immune to weight bias, their experience is usually different from that of female-identified people. Men are typically under less pressure to conform to a certain body shape; this is not to say the pressure doesn't exist, but that it is often easier for men to compensate for it in social settings. Certainly, fat men are as likely to be thought of as lazy or slovenly as women, but they are less likely to be openly harassed or attacked for it. The most obvious reason for this is that a big part of women's purpose as social creatures is to be attractive. Though the pressure on men is growing (plastic surgeries on men have skyrocketed in the last couple years, for example) we have a ways to go before men's appearances become their most powerful social tool, as is often the case for women. Women's appearances actually have measurable effects on their lives beyond simply feeling unattractive; fat women are statistically less likely to attend college, and make less money than their thinner counterparts, who are themselves making less money than men of all sizes. This is tied up with socioeconomic class, certainly, but it's also true that it's related to the fact that fat women as a group are more likely to fail in one of the most important tasks our culture expects a successful woman to complete: that is, being feminine.

Being feminine and being femme are two very different concepts. "Feminine" is the default gender presentation for women in the US. Fashion magazines, television, movies, books, and pop music all contribute to the lifelong education of women on how to be feminine. The feminine body is the one we often rail against, the one that's necessarily slender but not too slender, muscular but not too much so, hairless, poreless, graceful, beautiful, apologetic, and reluctant to take up space.

Femmeness, however, is interrogated femininity. Femmeness is femininity dragged through some mud, kicked in the stomach, given a good scrubbing, teased into a bouffant, doused in glitter, and pushed onstage in search of a spotlight. At least, this is how I define it. You will find as many definitions of femme as there are femmes to supply them. The concept of femme originated within LGBTQ communities as a means of differentiating those who choose to adopt a gender expression that employs certain aspects of traditional femininity in a performative and playful way. The main thrust of the idea is that femmeness is not a faithful reproduction of the feminine, but is instead a reinvention, reclamation, or ironic performance of it, taking place outside the traditional context of a misogynist world. I've known many a fat femme in my life who has felt a strong kinship to the concept of drag, and I would argue that all variations of feminine costume are drag—just some kinds of drag are more culturally acceptable than others. So, from my perspective, the "elephant in drag" is not altogether an unpleasant or inaccurate notion, though I do understand why it might cause others distress.

Several years ago, I gave up pants. The truth is, I've never been fond of pants. Finding pants that fit was an exercise in absurdity. I spent years tirelessly searching for an object that did not exist. I was fully aware that it did not exist, and yet I was compelled to seek it out nonetheless. I flirted with living a pants-free lifestyle for a long time before committing to it fully: every so often I'd believe in pants again, and would make an ill-advised purchase from Old Navy or Lane Bryant, but every single attempt ended in tears. So finally I gave them up. I quit pants. "Pants," I said, "you are fired. Get out of my office."

When I was a graduate student with a surplus of time and creativity, I made most of my skirts. They were skirts in bright and vivid tones, made of yards upon yards of fabric, full and dramatic, ending precisely at mid-knee, and often featuring strange appliqués I devised: giant eyeballs, a huge, fuzzy peach, cheerful-looking ants parading along the hem. Obviously, these were not the sort of skirts that I could find in stores, and not merely because of my size. If I were to call myself a mediocre seamstress, it'd be a tremendous compliment, but never underestimate a stubborn fat lady's desire for a collection of really strange skirts to motivate her to learn to make that one garment extremely well. My skirts were not particularly feminine, and were most often worn with battered Dr. Martens boots and striped tights. I had spent most of my life thus far convinced that I had no right to the trappings of traditional femininity simply because I was fat. This idea impeded my access to the cultural markers that might have helped me become the feminine ideal I thought I was supposed to be, and so while I may be wearing skirts, they would be the oddest skirts you ever saw.

Clothing is a language, for better or worse. Each garment carries an encoded meaning, woven directly into the fabric between the warp and weft. A suit may assert professionalism, or seriousness, or an association with a certain job or socioeconomic class. A skirt may demonstrate youth, or sensuality, or modesty. When we dress ourselves, even when we are doing so not for the purpose of drawing attention, we are sketching out what we want to say to people who see us every day, people with whom our interactions are only as deep as the fabric we wear. These interactions are ubiquitous enough to simply ignore, if you like, barring the occasional compliment, or harassment.

Dressing to be ignored is not a tremendous challenge, even for fat people. We are encouraged to disappear. Most of what is available in larger sizes tends to be loose fitting (the better to obscure our shapes) and unremarkable (the better to blend into the visual background noise of life). There is little access to attention-grabbing fashion for fatasses. What does this say about how fat people—and fat women in particular—are expected to dress? Fat bodies should be rendered as unobtrusive and as ignorable as possible; visibility is a privilege that must be earned by strict adherence to the established standards of appearance. When fat people dress in ways that encourage people to look, it is in direct violation of these ideas, and very often we wind up reaping a whirlwind of responses.

Picking through the terrible plus-size selection at my local Target one day, I was dimly aware of two teenage girls chatting with a third, a store employee on fitting room duty, a few yards away. Within moments their whispers, giggles, and confidential glances at me—though not at my face—made plain that I, possibly in combination with my outfit, was the subject of their shared humor. It was really the dress, I suspect, as the dress I was wearing thoroughly flouted the conventions of what is flattering for a person of my size to wear, with its three-tiered ruffled skirt making my hips and ass look dramatically, even comically, enormous. I often favor clothing that fucks with proportion, that makes me look bigger still in some respect, building upon the bigness of my actual body. On a political level, wearing such things is a kind of silent activism foisted upon everyone who has the fortune to see me that day; on a personal level, I just like ruffles.

I tried to ignore them, but the giggles went on, as though the girls believed me to be not merely extremely fat and curiously dressed, but also stupid or maybe hard of hearing. Few things disarm me as completely as teenage girls. I am heroically unfazed by the harassment of teenage boys, but girls are another matter. Boys are down for a confrontation: they yell, I yell back, or laugh, or crack a joke, and we both go on about our lives with very little lingering anger. The harassment of teenage girls tends to rely more on quiet humiliation, whispers behind cupped hands, comments delivered with a deceptive smile. There is no call and response; there is no give and take. If I am with a friend, I may respond by whispering and giggling as well, but on my own, there are few things I can do that won't escalate the circumstances, when usually I don't want that at all. I just want them to stop.

Possibilities ran though my mind. I could say: "Hey girls, what's so funny?" Or "A word of advice: you may want to be more subtle with your mockery, otherwise you look like assholes." Or "Excuse me ladies, can I ask your opinion? Which of these two dresses do you think is more likely to get me whispered about and laughed at?" The risk of speaking something aloud, however, is that although I imagine myself calmly asking about the humiliation factor of a garment, it is far more likely that my voice, once loosed, will only issue forth a string of abusive profanity while I'm shaking with rage. So I tend to say nothing.

Instead I circled around the rack between us and stood in full view of the group, feigning interest in an ugly tunic. I looked up and smiled, forcing myself to make eye contact with each girl in turn. I had intended it to be as sincere a smile as I could manage—a kill-them-with-kindness approach—but it came out wrong and rapidly resolved itself into a sneer. I stood and gamely stared black-bladed daggers at the three girls, all of whom had been facing my direction. One, after a moment of looking very uncomfortable, turned her back to me. Another kept glancing up to see if I was still glaring. I was. They were silent, their body language stiff and uncomfortable. *Is this weird for you? I thought. Is being openly stared at and judged by a total stranger weird for you? Do you fail to enjoy it?* I was seething. *All I am trying to do here is browse this preposterous collection of plus-size clothing and you girls, you feel entitled to stand there and laugh.*

Though I was still angry—and I allow myself anger, in these situations, as anger is healthier than internalizing shame—I also felt a kind of sympathy. Girls of that age are rarely kind. They don't know. They don't know that fifteen years into the future they could be on the other end of this exchange. They see things from one perspective and in one direction only. Seeing me so willfully and pointedly sticking out in that world is a disaster too challenging to process. Were their points and giggles because they assume I stand out only because I don't know better? Probably. The concept of standing out on purpose is not a familiar trope to many people of any age. Why would anyone do that? Why would I go out in public like that and make myself . . . a target?

I do it, in part, because others do, and because I want to support their efforts. I also want to show others that they can do it too. Standing out is okay. Standing up is okay. Doing both at once, well, that's activism. Those Target girls can laugh at me for having the gall to look out of the ordinary, and I can know it comes from a place of insecurity and immaturity and, probably, a sense of not-fitting-in-ness of their own. Curiously, that knowledge makes me want to stand out *more*. I'm educating you kids; you don't even know it.

Fatshion—fat + fashion—is a means of increasing visibility.

That said, for those of us who struggle against a lack of access to dress ourselves in interesting and attention-grabbing ways, this is not our primary motivation. The benefits that fatshionable style confers upon the individual are numerous and are often compelling enough to make the broader body politics merely flutter along behind, like the tail of a kite. Fashion can make us feel good about ourselves, especially in social situations. There is a measureable boost to your self-confidence when you walk into a crowded room wearing something that makes you feel like the hottest shit that ever walked into any crowded room anywhere. If you've ever owned a dress, a suit, a pair of jeans, or any other garment that had this effect, you know what I mean. You are unstoppable, you are magic. This is the movie version of the moment in your life when you walk into the party and everyone turns to look in rapturous awe, their gazes drawn from every corner as they can sense the gravity of your fabulousness and it is irresistible.

This may not actually happen. But the garment makes us believe it will, because it makes us feel as though our very best qualities are on display—be those qualities physical or intellectual or both. It is enough that the dress makes us feel good; we don't always have to be also fixated on the long-term effects of fat visibility. Simply taking action by standing out is often activism enough. It doesn't require a blaring soundtrack.

As much as fatshion choices may mean to the individual, they represent even more when drawn out into public discourse. Culturally speaking, participation in fashion in the first place represents how we care for ourselves, and that we care for ourselves at all. The successful application of style to a fat body can mitigate many of the negative assumptions people will inevitably make about that fat person. This is useful to know, especially when faced with circumstances in which "making up" for one's fatness is a necessity, and in which being radical is not an option. This is why we wear suits to job interviews. This is why we pull out our most "flattering" dress for a first date.

The drawback is that while we can use fashion as a

back-door method of confronting prejudice, this also results in massive pressure for fat people to be extra put-together, all the time, to be respectable fatasses, to stand in opposition to those unacceptable fat people, the ones who wear sweatpants and shirts with grease stains on them. You know them. The ones who make fat people look bad, like every stereotype is deserved, like we really are the disgusting horrors that we're made out to be.

There is something inhuman about a stereotype—that's the point. Negative stereotypes operate to remove the personhood of the stereotyped group, to make it difficult, if not impossible, for anyone to relate to them on a human level. On the one hand, sweatpants and shirts with grease stains are a statement no matter who is wearing them. Their message is, "I don't care about how I'm dressed right now." The "right now" is important because one cannot always assume that a person who runs to the corner store in sweatpants and a soiled shirt necessarily dresses that way all the time. If the person wearing the clothing is otherwise slender and attractive, we're usually willing to imagine the reasons why: maybe she's sick, or maybe she's in the middle of writing a term paper, or maybe she's doing laundry. She must have a reason. But when it happens to be a fat person who is sloppily dressed, the stereotype kicks in: the sweatpants and stained shirt represent not only a disregard for fashion at a given moment in time, but a systematic failure to adhere to the most common standards of appearance. A fat person is believed to have little respect for her appearance in the first place, simply by virtue of being fat, so she cares nothing for fashion, and of course she has no regard for the tender eyeballs of those other individuals upon whom she foists her sweatpanted, stained fattery in public. She is a visual—and even moral—disgrace.

Yet, she also may be sick, or writing, or doing laundry. And even if she's not, even if she is simply a person not much interested in fashion, she should have the right to step out into public, fat and sloppily dressed, and not be forced to face candid disgust from strangers. What is she doing wrong? How is she hurting anyone? She may offend our delicate sensibilities but ultimately there is no real damage done, except to our expectation that people who fail to meet cultural standards of attractiveness should not offend our sight in public, that we should be protected from having to look at them.

The pressure on fat people to go above and beyond in terms of appearance and presentation is much higher than it is on the non-fat population—the fats have far more to overcome, after all. When you further complicate this pressure with those associated with other marginalized groups, it becomes an incredible burden. For example, fat black women have added pressures to maintain a respectable appearance because they face expectations stemming from both racist stereotypes and from size-based ones. The concept of respectability itself is intrinsically tied with race, as is the idea of uplifting a marginalized group by presenting oneself in ways that aspire to be more mainstream, or, to put it plainly, more white.

When I was working toward my first master's degree, I had a professor describe the difference between liberal feminism and radical feminism in terms of pie. She stated that liberal feminists are asking for their share of the pie, a piece as big as anyone else's. However, radical feminists are asking for a different pie altogether. Liberal activism (i.e., "We're just like you!" activism) tends to be a conversation about assimilation and tolerance, and about being given a place at the table. Radical activism sees the existing system as broken and unsalvageable, and attempts to subvert, if not destroy the system altogether.

Thus, a radical fat activist approach to the question of access to clothing (and thereby respectability) might opt out of participation in the retail clothing world altogether, relying instead on producing one's own clothing, or by patronizing independent designers and small businesses that cater expressly to larger bodies. Radical fatshion activists might also choose to wear clothing considered to reinforce negative stereotypes as a political statement: even a muumuu can be a powerful icon of fat politics.

F requently I get compliments from much slimmer people, usually women, on my clothes, or on my style in general. Compliments are always lovely to hear, and they can also be deeply satisfying, considering the time and effort I put into my wardrobe. But there's also an aspect of these compliments that's, well, frustrating. Because when a much slimmer person compliments my clothing, she doesn't fully comprehend what she's complimenting.

I have known many non-fat people in my life, and have borne witness to their shopping travails. In my experience, non-plus-size shopping happens in a different world compared to the shopping I do. Straight-size shopping involves traveling to the nearest mall, going into several shops, trying stuff on, making vague complaints about fit or fabric, and eventually finding some degree of success, insofar as making a purchase. There are setbacks, there are petty frustrations. Sometimes things are unflattering. Sometimes current styles are not suited to personal tastes. These are certainly annoyances, but overall it is a fairly straightforward procedure.

Not so with the plus-size shopping experience. I'll use myself as an example. In US women's sizes, I wear size twenty-two to size twenty-eight, inclusive. Yes, this is a broad range of sizes, but it must be when you're trying to fit a non-standard body into a standard set of measurements, especially when that set of measurements can vary dramatically—and unpredictably—from one store to the next.

So I may begin at the mall too. If I'm very fortunate, there will be more than one store there that carries sizes large enough for me to try on. If not, I'll have to go to another mall, which may or may not have shops that carry my size. I may even have to go to a third mall before I can find a reasonable selection of clothes big enough just to try on. Of course, given that I'm in the US, the store is likely to be Lane Bryant and I tend to hate everything at Lane Bryant, no matter the season or the trends.

Having met with splendid failure at the mall, I will now go home and start shopping online, which is where I purchase the overwhelming majority of my clothing anyway. In this case, let's say I shop at four websites, and consult four different sizing charts, and squint intensely at numerous online images, trying to discern the hand of the fabric or how roomy the sleeves are or whether the waistline has elastic in it. I place two orders and pay shipping twice.

Then I wait.

Days later the packages arrive. Hooray! It's like Christmas. Of course, odds are good that the majority of what I've ordered will not fit or will fit badly. Returns will require paying shipping a second time in most situations. By the end of the experience, I may have lucked out with one or two items that I like, and that fit, but they cost me markedly more than the same clothes available in straight sizes, took over a week to receive, and I've lost money on the items I've had to return in the giant robber-baron casino that is plus-size online shopping.

And somehow, I manage to go through life without murdering anyone in a fit of fashion-deprived madness.

So whenever a not-fat person compliments my clothing, I get that they're saying, "You have great taste!" I appreciate it. I do. But I also occasionally feel like explaining, "You're complimenting me assuming that I just walked into a store one day and bought this because it appealed to me, like you do, and that it is my taste which is the impressive and compliment-worthy thing. No. In fact, it is my persistence in the dogged pursuit of decent fucking clothing that fit me that you should be complimenting. It is my ferocious tenacity in hunting for discounts, deals, and dragging heretofore unknown plus-size options from the caves of fatshion obscurity into the sunlight as a normal part of my endless hunt for fat style. I SLAYED A FUCKING DRAGON BEFORE I COULD BUY THIS DRESS. THAT IS WHAT YOU SHOULD BE COMPLIMENTING."

Instead I just say, "thank you." And I smile.

As good as we may feel when we've succeeded—slaying the dragon and making ourselves noticeably fatshionable—fashion also has the capacity to make us feel terrible about ourselves. Fat bodies that are left out of fashion are also left out of the larger conversation of style and personal expression taking place in the public sphere. Trying to express ourselves using a limited set of resources is like trying to talk with one-third of a full vocabulary—you can do it, but the subtleties are going to be lost. Not being able to participate in this conversation can be socially isolating, both insofar as being prevented from engaging in the ritual of shopping and from being fully seen.

Though fatshion is often possible, it is not always practical. Many people do not have the financial resources to invest in a thoughtfully assembled wardrobe. Others have limited plus-size shopping options because of where they live. Further, this is work that requires time and energy—how much of both do I expend in shopping? I hate to think about it. I may have that luxury, but many people do not. More than that, no one should be forced to care about clothing and style, lest we fall back into the oppressive notion that fat people have a responsibility to be *extra* put-together, to be *extra* meticulous in their dress and presentation in order to compensate for their unacceptable size. Fatshion should be fun, not a source of anxiety and pressure.

Access is important. Demanding better options in the marketplace is important. Indeed, there are days when all I want is to be able to walk into a nearby shop and buy a simple pair of black tights in my size without having to place an order online and wait for the postal service to oblige me. While focusing on access may make success easier to measure, it does not change the cultural standards that make it difficult to be a fat person in this world in the first place. When we argue in favor of greater plus-size selection from a purely profit-based perspective by asserting to clothing manufacturers that they will make more money by increasing their range of sizes, we make that movement profit dependent. Which means, unfortunately, that if the manufacturers do not see the financial returns they hoped for, they feel no compunction about pulling the plus sizes.

The reward of improved access to plus-size fashion is not simply the freedom to spend one's cash on hot clothes, though that is a nice short-term benefit. The further-reaching reward is increased visibility. It's the growing capacity to be seen as fat people— to be recognized, not as dehumanized, headless bodies, but as multidimensional individuals who are, among other things, fat. Increasing our visibility is a first step toward changing cultural attitudes such that fat bodies are not seen as pathetic sources of pity or derision, but rather as just one more form that human diversity takes.

I believe that the movement to use fatshion to forcefully insert ourselves into mainstream culture happens in three stages: being seen, standing out, and getting loud.

Being seen is the passive form—the "baby steps," if you will—and as such tends to be a comfortable starting point. Fat people, women particularly, are told repeatedly from all corners that they do not deserve to be seen, that being seen is a "reward that must be earned by an unfaltering commitment to mainstream beauty standards." We are told that being seen is the right of those who diet and exercise, who otherwise put effort into meeting the ideal, surgically if necessary, even if the ideal can never be met. How often have you heard someone say of a non-slender woman in a too-tight skirt or a too-revealing blouse, "No one wants to see that"? Her insistence on being seen is practically an assault.

Standing out is an act of bravado. Like being seen, it fixates on public attention, but where being seen is a passive availability, standing out is a strong suggestion. Standing out requires courage, optimism, and a complete disregard for convention. It is a clear expression of activism: I weigh X pounds and I am wearing a miniskirt. My dress size is not carried by 90 percent of clothing stores but I am out in the world wearing something that fits.

Finally, being loud is a command. It shocks, and intentionally draws attention. It ensnares the gazes of strangers against their will—they cannot look away, in the classic sense of viewing a train wreck—even if they are horrified and disgusted by what they see. There is a point where that which terrifies us most becomes irresistible, even pleasurable. A fat body, dressed scandalously? We hate it, and we want it, and we hate that we want it. I don't care if you don't like it—you are going to look at it. You are going to see me. You have no choice.

These are the three modes of the radical fatass.

Our bodies are signal towers; the transmissions they send out are laden with information. They speak for us and depending on the context—depending on the viewer's assumptions—they may tell folks things that aren't true, things we must then correct. Our bodies are often mistaken for public property, but they are a mode of public discourse. Once you are awake to this, it becomes impossible to ignore.

Your body will draw attention. How you use it is up to you.

As a kid I often stymied my parents with my stubborn refusal to participate in whatever trends were rampant among my peers. More than that, I developed a habit of actively avoiding anything understood to be popular. One parent or the other would say, "Oh, is this what you kids are into," and I would recoil, aghast, wanting nothing to do with *what you kids are into*. I suffered a compulsion to distinguish myself, occasionally to my social detriment, but occasionally to my advantage. This was well in place by the time I reached high school.

A week or two prior to the start of classes my freshman year, I was to report to the school to be fitted for my uniform, which would then be ordered and delivered the first week. I was shifting, by choice, to a Catholic high school after spending my elementary and middle years in public institutions. The uniform concept was new to me. I found the idea thrilling, because I'd seen the movie *Girls Just Want to Have Fun* many times and imagined myself in Helen Hunt's brilliantly accessorized, transformable ensembles. I saw the uniform as a blank slate on which I could perpetrate all manner of subversion—of the uniform and of myself. I also saw it as a way to belong. It was deeply appealing, a creative challenge.

The fittings took place in two classrooms off the school cafeteria, one for boys, and one for girls. We stood in line until space opened in the appropriate classroom. It happened that the classroom where the girls' fitting took place would be where I'd attend my first theology class, required for all students, and where I'd be pleasantly scandalized by hearing the teacher say the word "fuck" (he was quoting from *The Blues Brothers*).

The uniform components were two pieces: a stiff, white, woven polyester, button-down shirt, with the school's initials in navy embroidery on the left front breast pocket; and an equally stiff, navy plaid, box-pleated skirt, with a button and zipper closure on the side. When my turn came, I found the room occupied by a number of girls quickly trying on an assortment of uniform pieces to determine what size to order. I approached a woman at the desk at the front of the room, who reached into one of the many open brown boxes behind her and handed me a shirt and skirt to try on, among the other nervous would-be freshman girls wrangling blouses and skirts over their civilian clothes, as fully undressing seemed out of the question. I attempted to put the blouse on over my T-shirt; it was too small. I pulled the skirt over my jeans: it wouldn't even button.

Sheepishly I brought them back to the desk. No one had asked us our sizes, but instead they looked us over as though we were cattle at auction and guessed based on what they saw. The woman handed me another shirt and skirt from another box. The shirt fit marginally better, buttoning up without trouble, though it was in retrospect brutally tight across my shoulders and upper arms. The skirt was still hopeless. I brought it back again, caught between feeling angry at being misjudged and embarrassed at being so apparently large. The woman mumbled something apologetic, her eyes on the order forms on the desk in front of her, and then she turned and dug through another box for a moment. Eventually she waved me toward the boxes stacked two high beside the desk, bursting with chaotic heaps of discarded white poplin and navy plaid and said, "See if you can find something that fits." I don't remember her actually speaking to me before this point, I just remember she handed me garments without making eye contact.

I went into the boxes and dug. Too small, too small, too small. Everything was far too small and I knew it. It seemed the blouse I'd been given was the largest size they had. Though now I regret not demanding they order me blouses in the next size up, at the time I was still a true believer in the power of numbers, so I was simply relieved to (technically, if not comfortably) fit into a blouse marked as a sixteen and not require special consideration. As I pulled out skirt after skirt looking for anything larger than a twelve, I felt my panic rising. At this point in my life I'd spent a few years buying the largest size in the straight-size store, even when it was so tight as to be painful, because in

1990, succumbing to plus sizes would have been Style Death, my only options a Lane Bryant a thousand times more matronly and shapeless than today (if such a thing is even fathomable), or the abysmal torment of mail-order catalog doom. If avoiding that fate meant having to lie on my bed and breathe deep in order to zip up my size eighteen jeans from Lerner's, then so be it. But here, in the terrible land of unforgiving woven polyester uniforms, what if the largest size wasn't an option? Inside my head I couldn't even conceive that larger sizes than those represented in these boxes existed. I imagined myself being turned away from the school simply because they didn't make a uniform skirt to fit me.

Finally, at the bottom of a box, neatly folded and untouched by teenaged-girl hands prior to my own, I found a skirt marked eighteen. I grabbed at it like a drowning man clutches a life preserver and unfurled my plaid victory, waving it like a flag to the rest of the room, which, fortunately, ignored me. It didn't matter if it didn't fit now; I would figure out a way to make it work. Pulled over my jeans, buttoned and zipped, it was gasp-inducingly tight at the waist but I didn't care. Triumphant, I brought my too-tight blouse and too-tight skirt back to the desk where the women were filling out the order forms. I would bring that particular set home with me that day, as everyone did, to have a uniform to wash before the first day of school, when the rest of the ordered items would arrive. I ordered five too-tight blouses and three too-tight skirts.

Little did I know I would keep and wear those same blouses and skirts for four whole years. The blouses were so tight in the arms it was difficult for me to reach forward and down to pick up a pencil if I dropped one on the floor. The unyielding fabric kept my arms nearly immobile, except for a narrow range of movement. The skirts I would cherish because in my sophomore year the uniform code changed and the skirts were traded for culottes, and oh my friends, you cannot imagine the horror that is me, a butternut squash–shaped fat girl, in knee-length plaid culottes. Those of us with skirts from the prior year were allowed to keep wearing them, and thus I treasured my waist-constricting, breath-impairing skirts for the rest of my high school career.

A large part of my decision to attend private high school was rooted in my overwhelming social isolation in eighth grade. I believed that attending a private school instead of going on to the public high school with many of the same people who'd known me in middle school would give me a chance to reinvent myself. The uniform would seem, on the surface, to give me the option of blending in (if I felt so inclined) or standing out (if I was feeling my inner Helen Hunt). I thought of the uniform as a fresh sheet of paper on which I could write my identity every day. I thought of the uniform as a costume in which I could hide. But it failed. I was too awkward, too brainy, too big in multiple respects, to blend in, and I was still me, in a uniform or not. I was bursting at the seams—literally, figuratively, in every conceivable way.

Unfortunately, I would discover before long that the uniform did not eclipse style fads in the prevailing culture at school. In fact, it just narrowed the field. The axis on which the trends at my high school revolved was socks. Yes, socks. I learned rapidly that the correct socks were E.G. Smith slouch socks (which, astonishingly, have only recently been discontinued by the manufacturer). These were cotton socks that came in many colors (including tie-dye) and were meant to intentionally bag loosely around one's ankles, not unlike legwarmers. Because they had no elastic at all, by day's end one's E.G. Smith socks often slumped over the back of the heel to drag on the ground, which made keeping the lighter colors clean a challenge. The inventive could fashion sock garters from standard rubber bands, hidden by folding over a narrow cuff at the top of the sock, which many of us did. These pretentious socks were also criminally overpriced. As I recall, on back-to-school shopping trips in high school at the late lamented Florida-exclusive department store Burdines, the social status afforded by a single pair of these name-brand socks would cost you between $12 and $14 (tie-dye was more expensive) in 1990.

So I bought some of these ridiculous socks, with the vivid "love, eric" printed in gold ink on the sole, to identify them as the real thing and not some knockoff. And I wore them, briefly, to see how it felt to fit in. Except it didn't work. I still never felt like I fit in, even in a school uniform, even with the correct socks, even dressed like everyone else.

It wasn't long before I'd cast aside my E.G. Smith socks in favor of odd legwear collected from clearance bins and discount stores: patterned knee-highs, fishnet anklets, anything that spoke the opposite of the giant, cotton slouch socks that everyone else seemed to covet and favor. Because it seemed to me, even in those hoary teenage years of trying to figure out who I was, that a sizable part of being myself meant standing as a contradiction to popular convention. It meant being not just *willing*, but *compelled* to be visibly different as a counterpoint to the norm, accepting the abuse as well as the admiration that a life of even subtle subversion seems to attract.

At sixteen I decided that nearly everyone who went to my high school was terribly boring, not least because no one seemed to know about the music I liked and music was the single most important thing in my life at the time. Once I recognized a guy from my class in the mosh pit at a Bad Religion show, but when I approached him at school the following day I received a devastating dismissal. Was I so uncool? Or was it because I was, at the time, the fattest girl in our whole high school? Fuck him. I was searching for someplace different to belong anyway.

I discovered the Hot Moon Café through a guy named Jason I had met on the internet. The Hot Moon was a DIY-styled coffeehouse, ramshackle and improvised like something a clutch of displaced bohemians might have assembled via dumpster-diving while squatting in a strip mall. At the time it was the most perfect place on earth, an oasis of invention and acceptance where all sorts of local musicians, poets, artists, and other experimenters could assemble and be relatively assured that no one would laugh at them or their efforts—at least not out loud. This isn't to suggest that everyone there was talentless or a hack; that would be inaccurate. But we *were* very young. Most of us, certainly I can speak for myself, didn't really know what we were doing.

Wednesdays were open mic nights. I read poetry. I read embarrassing, self-righteous high school poetry. And there's more: I sang. A friend played guitar so I could sing The Murmur's "You Suck" as loudly as possible, and the occasional Violent Femmes song. I wanted to be a certain person. I wanted to stand on a stage and demand the attention of an audience, to have them listen and hear me, not to see me as a tragic fat girl but as a person who was interesting.

It was at Hot Moon that I impulsively kissed a boy I didn't know in front of a table full of people, over a game of Jenga. It was a wildly out-of-character moment. A friend who was present pulled me aside to ask "What the hell was that?" I didn't know. I just felt like doing it. I later dated that boy and like every other boy I dated as a teenager, he was gay. There was another boy, a year or two older, who would hug me whenever we saw each other, pressing my body into his, his hand in the small of my back, not in a creepy way but with kindness and appreciation—and I thought, "Huh."

At twenty, during a sexual encounter my partner mumbled, "I love your body," and I was immediately distracted by this, not the "I love" part, but "your body." For the first time ever, I realized I have a body. What I mean is, I never thought of myself as simply having a body. I had an albatross, a mistake, a burden. But then, for the first time, I realized I have a real body, just as it is, no matter what it looks like.

I fell in with the goth scene in Boston, where I was an undergrad. Unlike South Florida where I grew up, Boston was home to a thriving subculture. And although I doubted my place within it—always held back by my belief that I was not cool enough to be goth—the key, of course, was community. We all rejected the cultural norms and survived together.

There is often a protective impulse in subcultures, automatic and kneejerk, because most everyone in that community is accustomed to being harassed or treated as an outsider. I used to go to Manray, a club in Cambridge. We would take public transportation in big groups because it was the only way to go and be relatively safe from the harassment we regularly received from random people on the train, our sartorial choices an open invitation for scorn. We were all in black, wrapped in fishnet, much of our clothing improvised, and it's not Halloween, you know? The alternative, if you missed traveling with the group, was to go to the club in "normal" gear and change once you got there.

The goth club was the first environment in which I saw fat women being beautiful and sexy, wearing clothes I never would have considered possible, and getting positive and appreciative attention from others. I ran into a lot of bog-standard chubby chasers (known also as "fat admirers") at the goth club—straight men who are quietly queered by their attraction to fat women, and who seek out subcultural spaces where no one judges their proclivities. On the one hand, their interest made me uncomfortable because very often it was purely physical, and though there is nothing wrong with purely physical interest, it was often objectifying in a way that I personally found off-putting. But it was also proof that it is possible to be attracted to a fat body, which is a preference portrayed as either impossible or pathological in most mainstream cultural circumstances.

In some queer communities, there are spaces, albeit not always positive ones, for attractions to fat bodies. In straight circles, such spaces rarely exist and the ones that do are driven deep underground, which only reinforces the notion that to be attracted to a fat body is something shameful, dirty, and wrong.

In the 1994 film *Muriel's Wedding*, Toni Collette plays Muriel Hesslop, a socially inept fat woman living in a provincial town in Australia where she is surrounded by her old school friends—"friends" only insofar as they begrudgingly allow Muriel to spend time with them while they ignore or abuse her. Whereas Muriel is awkward and not conventionally attractive, her friends are slender, tanned, and cocksure. Near the beginning of the film, there is a scene in which a cheerful Muriel joins her friends at a bar and learns that they are going on holiday without her. While she's still processing this, Muriel's friends inform her that they no longer want her to be part of their social group. By way of explanation, they argue that Muriel is fat, does not know how to dress, and is generally embarrassing. When Muriel, crestfallen and pathetic, agrees, "I know I'm not normal, but I'm trying to change. I'm trying to become more like you . . . " They assure her, with barely concealed disdain, "You'll still be you."

After a few moments of silence, during which the group turns its attentions to other matters, Muriel bursts into tears, sobbing noisily, wheezing for breath, and drawing the attention of the other people in the bar. She explodes, "I'm not nothing! I'm not nothing," while her friends physically recoil. Muriel feebly argues for her personhood to these women who really do see her as nothing, disposable, an unwanted hanger-on. But even Muriel, who still wants to be included in spite of their poor treatment, can't swallow the notion that she is less than a person for failing to fit in with the pretty-party-girl archetype represented by the rest of the group.

It doesn't phase them that Tania, recently married and therefore representative of the greatest success, has been alternately weeping and shouting throughout this exchange, expressing her sorrow and rage at having discovered that her new husband has cheated on her. This theatrical pain from the group's de facto leader is a cue for the rest of the group to stroke and soothe, to listen and reassure. In contrast, Muriel's pain is unseemly. Her sobs are anguished, her face flushed bright red, her blubbering incoherent and desperate. Muriel is what we would call in the vernacular an "ugly crier."

Muriel's pain is long buried and intricately woven into her whole identity, the product of an abusive parent and a profound lack of self-esteem. She lies compulsively when we first meet her, making up a life she doesn't have, trying desperately to fit in to a world that does not recognize her value (if only because neither does she). Muriel insists that she is "not nothing." The society she longs to be part of not only rejects her but *erases* her. Muriel still tries to fight back.

Our cultural ideology of beauty-as-personal-responsibility contributes to a world in which all bodies are public property, open to criticism, compliment, or mockery, at all times. There is no line drawn between the faux perfection of models in ads and the real bodies of women going about their lives—we are all expected to strive for the impossible, no matter what it takes, and when we refuse, our subversion is punished by social censure.

A mismanaged body, or rather, a body that is perceived as mismanaged, is a thing to be feared. The overly cared-for body—one that is too obviously embellished with cosmetics and plastic surgery, one that is too meticulous in how it eats or moves, one that is guarded or coddled or fabricated so that the seams are still visible—is as much a source of discomfort and pity as one that seems not to be cared for at all.

It takes effort, often a great deal of effort, in order for the vast majority of human bodies to fall in line with the perfectionist ideologies of beauty as they are put forth in media imagery, always photoshopped into the realm of impossibility. However, the work one does isn't supposed to show; this undertaking should be an invisible one. Beauty should be effortless—"natural"—

and the cross one bears in order to achieve it should be minimized lest the fixation become unseemly. Nobody wants to believe that beautiful women must martyr themselves to that cause; nobody wants to know how much they sacrifice in the service of their appearance. We prefer to think of these efforts as mysterious, alchemical formulas shared in hushed tones, treasure maps to the source of natural attractiveness: "beauty secrets."

When beauty takes too much work, it is perceived as desperate, even pathetic. Muriel Hesslop works hard, so very hard to fit in with her pretty friends, but the harder she tries the uglier she becomes, and it's only when she has given up on being someone else that we see her as she really looks—first thing upon waking, without makeup, having decided to go home and to bring her compulsive lies to a definitive end. In this moment, Muriel is beautiful, not because of her face, but because of her understanding that she has value, even without fitting in, without being "normal."

Beauty standards are so unpredictable that they cannot even be rightly referred to as a code—a code could be cracked. If fat exists in the service of sexualizing a body, it is sometimes okay: yes to fat tits, fat hips, within reason, a fat ass, depending, though it cannot be too fat or too rugged. If the skin is poreless and taut then you are probably in business. Other fat is never acceptable: fat bellies, dimpled knees, a crease at the ankle or wrist. Bodies that are too fat all over are a problem, certainly. So are bodies that are shaped "wrong"—all belly, no ass, small-breasted, too short, flesh that folds at knees and elbows, a line of cleavage that runs too long or crookedly, chins that double or triple with the application of a smile or laugh—as well as bodies that function "wrong"—a lack of strength, a lack of mobility, an impaired sensory perception, too feminine, too masculine, not feminine enough, not masculine enough, a bad knee, a bad back, a bad autoimmune system, a brain firing on different pathways.

There have been periods in history in which thinness was reviled, viewed as a sign of failure or sickness much as fatness is today. These standards are arbitrary, and being arbitrary they are only meaningful because of the significance our culture assigns to them. If we valued large bellies and flat asses, these different standards, refreshing though they may seem now, would continue to oppress those without these attributes. The bodies we do not value, we fear. Fear comes in many flavors and the revulsion with which we're taught to regard these deviant bodies is a variant of fear. It's a fear of the unknown, of these strange forms, which we do not see, which we have not been taught to read. We have no context in which to parse them.

Most of us spend our lives steeped in this mire of idealized figures. Mass-produced images are the reason we have a visual frame of reference for an idealized body. Prior to the proliferation of this media, the only points of reference we had were our families and immediate communities. In reality, different bodies look, move, and function in different ways and difference itself ought not to be a source of shame. Yet cultural beauty standards seem hell-bent on erasing the unique quirks of these individual differences in favor of one body, one face, one skin tone, one ideal. One single point of comparison for us all.

There are exceptions, of course. Some people have made special efforts to expand the range of bodies that they can see and appreciate. This requires a plan, an intention, a stubborn push, and it still does not fully insulate us.

Every once in awhile the fashion world will suddenly embrace the speciously named "plus-size models" and these women are immediately everywhere, usually naked, the running joke being that there are no sample sizes to fit them. But the nakedness is purposeful, because these soft bodies are edgy, so unlike the standard forms we see in popular culture. Crystal Renn, arguably the most successful and recognizable plus-size model in recent memory, told the *New York Times*, "They see a roll, and they say, 'Ooh, a roll!' And they focus on it." It isn't diversity that the women's magazines and high-fashion auteurs are after; it's shock, amazement, attention, and a lot of self-congratulatory back-patting for their progressiveness and willingness to buck the oppressive norms that they themselves are responsible for shaping and enforcing. This body tourism is steeped in the language of beauty, advocating that *women of a certain size sure can be beautiful!* But of course there are limits—lest anyone think such occasional positive attention toward women who are slightly bigger than the norm for models is irresponsibly promoting self-esteem and self-acceptance, they are sure to remind us that "obesity is a significant health problem" and that these models aren't "obese" (except when they are, given that medical obesity actually looks far smaller than many of us may think).

The praise lavished on plus-size models is simply a matter of moving the goalposts; these women are marginally wider versions of the same idealized shapes to which we are accustomed. So we take a woman in the same style and increase the proportions. It's still the same body, just larger on the page.

Through mass media we learn to read all the shapes: a woman's body with large breasts, wide hips, and a narrow waist is typically going to be sexualized; a woman's body that is round all over is typically going to be portrayed as matronly. A woman's body that defies these expectations—say, a round-all-over body that is presented as sexualized—is disorienting and discomforting. Women perceived as too thin must constantly confront the assumption that their bodies are the result of starvation and irrational self-loathing and must assert that they eat, *they really do eat*, even as judgmental strangers instruct them on the value of sandwiches. This is no better than telling a fat person to put down the cake. Both are presumptuous and offensive. The reality is that all female-reading bodies are policed according to expectations of acceptability, femininity, and attractiveness. A body that is too skinny is read as fragile, delicate, frail; a body that is too fat is read as excessive, grotesque, expansive, perverse—and the fine lines between "too skinny" and "too fat" are murky domains whose precise borders are only in the mind of the beholder. In the middle ground of average size, there is no predicting these distinctions as they differ slightly depending on who is doing the looking.

I once discovered in my internet wanderings, among a cache of found vintage photographs, a full-length image of two women standing in a yard with the suggestion of a vine-wrapped trellis behind them. Their dresses are tea-length and belted, but otherwise loose fitting, worn with low heels, their hair pinned back. This picture was possibly taken in the late 1930s or early 1940s. The woman on the right seems past middle age, given her posture, dress, and the tidy silk scarf encircling her neck. She wears a smile that is broad and genuine, lips parted, the skin around the eyes creased with frequent smiles past. The woman on the left smiles wanly, tight lipped, her jaw set, her discomfort palpable, with her hands clasped behind her back. Though her cheeks are still plump, she is more adult than child, in her late twenties perhaps, with full hips and bosom, and a not particularly defined waistline. I would not call her fat, though neither is she slender. Is she the daughter of the woman on the right, or her niece or friend? As a found photograph, we will never know. All we know is what someone has written on the back of this picture: "I just have to quit eating and work hard."

Women have been quitting eating and working hard for decades with little to show for it. Women's body hatred is cyclical, and fat people have always existed, so it is not surprising that examples of women's troubled relationships with their appearance can be found throughout our photographic history. The words on the back of this photograph are not a prescription for a future generation—they are firmly lodged in the moment, a recrimination, a note to the woman from herself: *Do you see what you really look like? This is what you must do to fix it.* The woman in the image, who wrote those words, is likely no longer alive, and I wonder whether in her declining years she thought back on her life with regret, wishing she had spent more of it dieting.

On a 2010 family trip to Disney World, we hooked up the digital camera to the resort television one evening and paged through the pictures we had taken that day. In one photo, one female family member looked at herself and exclaimed, with some degree of horrified astonishment, "Am I *really* that fat?"

It's always a little odd, given that I am often one of the fatter people present in most social situations, to hear these sorts of inquiries and exclamations. The rest of the family launched into action with a chorus of, "No, of course not!" before I could formulate a more critical response of my own, but I continued to think about it. I am thinking about it even now. The image of ourselves that we carry around inside our heads is not always accurate: sometimes it is a fantasy body, a body we do not have, but the idea of which is more comfortable and familiar than the reality, which we rarely see from an objective perspective. Except in photographs.

The explosive "Of course not!" is part of the social script; it is the anticipated response. This is, in fact, the pivot on which most casual conversations about fatness revolve. A person asks, "Do I look fat in this?" The script demands we say no. Anything less would be cruel. A person states, "I am so fat and disgusting!" The script demands we argue and soothe. A person cannot be allowed to go on believing she is fat. Even when she is.

In American culture in particular, there is an inextricable link between *any* photograph of a fat body, no matter the context, and the archetypal "before" picture, the one we have seen our whole lives as advertisements for weight loss. The examples of photo-shock described above are hardly unique; we've all heard them before, from friends and strangers alike, from people who were sailing merrily through life, totally unaware of how unhappy they're supposed to be because of how they look. You have probably experienced it yourself. One day you see an unflattering photograph of your body and, gasp, *THAT is how I really look?* And then, perhaps, *I have to DO something!*

Photographs still have to answer to the eye of the beholder. Pictures that I find unflattering, others do not, and vice versa. This is how it goes. Because so many of the images we see on a daily basis are saturated with perfect-seeming faces and bodies, many of which are achieved through digital manipulation, the expectation is that everyone can and should look that way. Photographs, frozen moments that they are, enable us to stop time and assess, and sometimes to admonish. We can fix on our flaws: *my breasts are uneven, my skin is too dark, my knees are ugly, my hair is disheveled, I look terrible.*

One diet book author who was moved to weight-loss salvation by an unflattering picture recommends that fat people get themselves photographed as a "reality check." See, lots of people with substandard bodies are walking around feeling happy a lot of the time, and that's a problem. Body culture tells us in no uncertain terms that fat people are not supposed to be happy; they are supposed to be ashamed. The notion of employing photography as a cure for happiness rests on the idea that seeing ourselves for the gargantuan monsters we really are will kill our lackadaisical contentment and eject us into a sad, dark void of self-loathing and body hatred, *where we belong.*

My parents brought me to the Olan Mills photography studio, where I smiled and glowed, a toddler with perfect ringlets seemingly spun from sunlight itself (what happened to that hair?), wearing a frilly dress and shining patent leather mary janes. And then a year or so later, I sat myself with impeccable posture on a fake log, a two-dimensional forest behind me, my ankles crossed, knees apart, wearing shorts and a T-shirt emblazoned with a rainbow (dresses having become anathema), my hair stick-straight and shaped into the ubiquitous bowl cut of the era. Once I began school, I faced annual student portraits in which the photographer would invariably instruct me to "open your eyes more" when I smiled, advice that resulted in a few school pictures of me in an expression of bewildered madness. At some point I decided I did not like the space between my two front teeth, and so my smiles became tight-lipped and nervous. Eventually I devised a smile that parted my lips enough to look more natural, but not so much as to actually show the inside of my mouth. And this is the smile I wear in my high school senior portrait. The photographer handed me a black velvet "drape" in which I was to wrap myself, the same one all the girls used. It barely came up over my arms—in the final image the edges have slid down my shoulders, my bra straps photoshopped away.

I had a judicious and obsessive consciousness of how I appeared in these photographs. I felt a compelling need to control my image in a literal way. In my current driver's license picture I am half-smiling that same tense closed-mouth smile of my middle adolescence, though for years I did not smile at all. By thirty-two I had developed a certain comfort with self-portraits; I chronicled my outfits on a near-daily basis for online fashion communities, but I had (have) yet to fully lose the urge to go rigid as a corpse when someone else points a camera in my direction.

A few years ago, I found myself being professionally photographed for the first time since childhood. The *Boston Globe* was set to run a profile of me as a major feature in their arts and living section, and they wanted a picture taken by a *Globe* photographer. I was rattled, but couldn't conceive of saying no. The experience involved over an hour of standing, leaning, hand clasping, hunching, dancing, reclining bemusedly on an antique sideboard (and lucky me it did not collapse), and twirling. The experience was uniquely exhausting.

I spent the time cultivating an acute awareness of every part of my body, and remembering to smile (with my eyes), while trying to keep all that concentration from showing in my face as the classically tense expression I have worn in photographs my whole life—*oh, I'm just having fun here, aren't I, and someone appeared with a very expensive camera to capture it.*

The photographer explained fairly early on in the shoot that the *Globe* does not retouch any of its photos ever. We had so many moments of exposure and whatever happened inside the camera's inner workings was what there was to work with. I felt both relieved and panicked by this information: relieved because I did not have to wrestle with the political discomfort of having my imperfections expunged, panicked because *but what about my imperfections? People will see them!*

The anxiety I felt between the end of the photo session and the publication of the article was something I had not endured in a long time. The experience required me to hand over control of my representation to someone else. It was sobering. For better or worse, photography has the power to influence our perception of ourselves. It'd been years since I'd looked at a picture of myself and given a mortified shiver upon failing to recognize the person there. I know what I look like and I am untroubled by it. The wonder of self-acceptance isn't that it makes you instantly attractive to everyone; it's that it makes you not care particularly whether other folks uniformly find you attractive or not. Too often body acceptance is inaccurately distilled into the idea that fat people just want other folks to find them pleasant to look at. No, but we would rather you not feel entitled to tell us how disgusting we are.

Our self-image rarely matches the image we're projecting in three dimensions, the person that others know. And why would it? That is not the perspective from which we are accustomed to seeing ourselves. Finding an image of ourselves unflattering or strange should be expected, because unless we are models or actresses, we are seeing our bodies from an unfamiliar angle. It does not mean we're in denial; it simply means we probably don't look at photos of ourselves very often, and this is easy enough to remedy.

The *Globe* used two photos of me—two very large photos—in the print edition of the article. In the picture on the section's front page, I am slightly bent forward, clasping my hands in front of me, frozen in mid-laugh. It is a joyful, exuberant picture. The picture inside is of me twirling and laughing again, and this one I like less because I fixate on the wrinkles in my dress. I can barely even see the rest of the picture, which others have complimented profusely, because all I see is that minor imperfection—*I should have ironed it better, or worn a different dress. Why didn't I wear black? Wrinkles barely show on black.* I didn't wear black because I didn't want to be the fat girl wearing black, because *it's slimming, you know.* I wanted to say "fuck slimming." I wanted to show my colors, a fat fucking butterfly caught mid-guffaw in the newspaper for all to see. Because I don't often see women who look like me in the newspaper, or in magazines, or on billboards not advertising bariatric surgery.

B y a serendipitous convergence of good fortune I live on a beach, and I have a balcony, on which I often sit during that brief period of the year when the weather in New England is pleasant enough to do so. From the beach I often hear conversations, car stereos, children shouting.

One morning I was sitting on my balcony, a book in my lap, when I heard a child's voice calling out, "Hey, ugly!" The sound rang a bell inside my head, as though the kid were shouting in my very ear, Hey, ugly. I felt a chill of panic, and every cell in my body seized as if struck by lightning.

I can't remember a period of my life in which I was not harassed by strangers, often for doing nothing more than existing. It has slackened with my age, as I grow more socially invisible, but given my predilection for loud dresses and my inability to be silent, I suspect it will always happen. My size will always make me a target. I am not surprised that a shout from an unseen child, and one likely not even directed at me as I was hidden behind a thick screen of plants, could affect me so.

School bus, high school, freshman year: a boy yelled, "That girl looks like a horse!" There was laughter. It happened often. I was called a name as if I were nothing, not real, an error, something that should have been discarded. I am not altogether certain the boy was even talking about me, but the people nearest to me assumed he was, given that I am fat, the natural target for abuse, the one who gave off victim-signals like a beacon. I slumped down the bus aisle in thinly disguised terror, every day—even my posture demonstrating my expectation that someone would assault me, because that was what I believed I was for, and of course, they obliged.

I never defended myself back then; I simply braced for impact. This was partly a practical matter. If I could find a way to receive the verbal onslaughts without being hurt by them, that seemed a more pragmatic approach than arguing with my attackers in favor of my right to be beautiful. Because even then I did not believe in any such entitlement. I knew, at fourteen, with an unshakeable certainty that I was not a pretty girl, no matter what well-intentioned family members might say, and that I never would be. Despite the fear there was a kind of freedom in that realization.

Seeing a woman on a reality television show speak of how her beloved made her "feel beautiful," my partner asked me, "Do I make you feel beautiful?"

This is a complex question and likely one I've never answered with complete accuracy. I told my partner, "I believe that *you* think I'm beautiful," and "You make me feel *loved*," both of which are true, but neither of which is the same as feeling beautiful myself. The fact of the matter is that I don't feel beautiful. Before you frown at this sympathetically, dear reader, allow me to note also that I don't feel as though I'm missing anything. My capacity (or lack thereof) to embody physical beauty is not a personal attribute that matters much to me. This is not to suggest that I do not appreciate beauty as a concept—I most assuredly do. However, while beauty is something I enjoy, it is not something I am inclined to be.

When my partner asks if I feel beautiful, I must say no, because I never feel beautiful by its strictest definition, because I am not a beautiful girl. I am rather a woman who knows where she stands, who feels comfortable and confident in her own skin, and yet who struggles daily with living in a world that tells her repeatedly that she shouldn't feel this way, that she has no right to feel this way. Our beauty, or our feelings of beauty, are often feelings we guard as ferociously as we would the most priceless treasure. We do this because for many of us, this feeling comes all too rarely.

Let's interrogate our assumptions: What do we really mean when we talk about feeling beautiful? We mean that we feel good about ourselves. We mean that we feel happy and confident and alive, and this combination of feelings is so rare and so magical and so intoxicating that we have to call it "beauty."

I can surrender the assumption that subjectively *feeling*—if not objectively *being*— beautiful in the conventional sense is a requirement of a happy and fulfilling life. Feeling beautiful should not be a critical aspect of all the big moments of our lives in the way that it is.

To use an obvious example, most married women I know felt enormous pressure to "feel beautiful" on the day they got married, as though the wedding would somehow fail to count if the beauty was missing. This is not to suggest that people shouldn't feel good about themselves as the occasion warrants, but this feeling should not be the necessity.

The danger of falling into the habit of demanding that our bodies—fat bodies, or otherwise "ugly" bodies—be pretty too is that by doing so we are reinforcing the cultural importance of prettiness. We are acknowledging a longing for social acceptance, a willingness to indulge prettiness pressures so long as we are allowed to play too. It is a classically liberal stance: all we want is our fair share.

I'd prefer to occupy a space outside the pretty/ugly paradigm, a space where the parameters are self-determined. Because I believe there is no circumstance in which these categories will not be oppressive, to someone somewhere. Because I want to reject that kind of system, not participate in it. The longing to appreciate and value oneself as a beautiful person is a fine notion. Confronting, deconstructing, and redefining what counts as beauty is a valiant effort. But we should also be vigilant: Is it personal gratification and self-love we're after, or the advantages that being beautiful to others would afford us?

No one should be forced to play the pretty game, though most of us born female spend our lives learning the rules and trying to get ahead. We are taught that we are not allowed to even consider removing ourselves from the playing field. And yet it is a game without end. Pretty is not an accomplishment to be won so much as a state of constant vigilance, even for women who qualify as beautiful in the cultural eye, because so many of these women still cannot see themselves as attractive. An intrinsic part of the pretty game is feeling inferior, imperfect, and incomplete. The players can compete, but no one can win.

Some years ago on a visit to my childhood home in South Florida, I sat on the floor of my father's home office (there was only one chair and he was in it) and walked him through the use of some program on his computer. I wore one of those girl-cut tees emblazoned with an angry-looking Hello Kitty from Hot Topic's new-at-the-time plus-size line, and jeans. We finished and as I stood up, my father blurted, almost like an explosion, apropos of nothing, "You've gained weight!"

I wasn't sure that this was true—the jeans I was wearing were a pair that I'd worn in high school, and they were bigger on me now, but I *was* wearing a shirt that didn't balloon over my body, as I traditionally had done. I presumed that his comment was based on being able to *see* me, as much as it was on any perceived change in my size. But it wasn't just the inaccuracy of the statement that got me. It was the tone. The words were delivered with a deeply unsettling mixture of astonishment and accusation. It ripped through me like a rusty blade. Yes, it did. And yet by this point I was lecturing to undergrads about media representation of women's bodies, and holding forth on fat acceptance in front of fifty students with nary a flutter of doubt. His words hit me like an unexpected wave, and carried me right back to my fifteenth year, to my dark bedroom. I'm listening to Tori Amos's "Silent All These Years" on the local indie radio station, my ear pressed against the speaker on the boom box, knowing that I could never be happy, that no one could ever truly love me, that I would always be disposable and disgusting and isolated until I lost enough weight.

I went into that old bedroom and closed the door. My partner was there. I sat on the bed, staring blankly at nothing, and he looked at me and asked, "What's wrong?"

I explained. He told me I had to say something. "I can't," I whispered. "I *can't!*" It was a still a whisper, but ferocious, certain. Those words wouldn't even form in my mouth. I couldn't tell my father that this hurt me. It was an impossibility. I may as well attempt to flap my arms and fly.

My partner would not let it go. He assured me repeatedly that it was a thing I was capable of speaking aloud. And if I was capable of speaking it, why would I keep it to myself? And yes, why not try? What would happen? Would I be struck mute? Would the language come out all garbled, like speaking in tongues? Would lightning hit me and pin me to the floor? Few of us manage to escape the desire to please our parents, to make them proud of us. We have to navigate the tricky straits of being true to ourselves and the people we want to be, while still feeling afraid that our choices might disappoint the people who raised us.

After a few minutes, I left the bedroom. I squared off in front of my unwitting father in the middle of the house. I told him that he had made a comment about my size and I needed to talk to him about it. And then I said, "You don't get to say that to me anymore."

I got as far as "don't" before my voice broke and I knew I wouldn't be able to avoid crying. I was embarrassed but let it go. And why not? Why hide that pain? Why bury it now? It was like the dam that had held it all back for so many years was failing, and instead of shoring it up, plugging the cracks, I brought my fist down and crushed the whole thing. I told my father that those comments hurt me, that they had always hurt me. I told him my body was not something he had a right to pass uninvited commentary on, and I didn't care that he was just trying to help when I was growing up as a fat kid who didn't want to be what I was. I knew his intentions were good; I knew he just wanted me to be happy. But it had damaged me. It had damaged me right down to my bones.

My father was shocked I suppose, but bless him, he tamped down any defensive impulses and listened. Or perhaps he was just too astonished to do anything else. He apologized. I didn't get into the nuts and bolts of body acceptance right then; it wasn't the time. I finished my piece and walked away. Back into my old bedroom. Back behind the closed door.

I felt, ironically, many pounds lighter.

I don't recall if I ever, aside from this moment, formally announced my intention to stop trying to lose weight to my family. But this interaction opened the door. It would be years before my family would accept my acceptance, and it would only come after extensive conversations about my weight, health, and happiness. It began because I stood up for myself for the first time, because I had a moment in which I couldn't sit by and quietly swallow my rage any longer. I think we all have this point, where the pressure builds and we have to open ourselves up and let it all fly free, as terrifying as it is to see our pain and rage spilled out into the air before us.

Anger is a natural response to the awareness that one has spent an uncertain amount of time, money, and attention on the pursuit of a potentiality that may not exist. Anger—sometimes mingled with despair—is often the first stop on the road to radicalness, and it's a detour you'll remember as a moment of magnificent discovery.

Oh, I remember when I was first outraged! I remember when the injustice of diet culture, of misogyny, of fascist, oppressive, and yet ubiquitous beauty standards was almost too much to bear, when I wanted to spend each day walking around carrying a hand-painted sign with some new nugget of wisdom printed upon it. In line at the grocery store: "Food is not the enemy." At the doctor's office: "Your body is not a tragedy." On the street, preempting the inevitable catcalls: "This is private property." Everywhere: "Fat and fuck you."

For some of us, the anger is borne of having spent so many years chasing the invisible unicorn of the perfect body—or rather, the body that is good enough for us to be satisfied with. This is an individual, personal, self-centered anger. Why didn't anyone tell me I was wasting my time—my life—believing what I was told, that I needed a certain (thin) body in order to be in love, go to Paris, wear dresses, feel beautiful and worthwhile and complete?

The anger can also be an obstacle. I have spent so long on the project of my body, I cannot give it up now, and I cannot deal with the suggestion that I should. So much energy wasted! Years ago, on one of those day-time talk shows that make me doubt the greater good of humanity, I saw a fat-acceptance activist on display in front of a studio audience of skeptics and nonbeliev-ers. Most questions were pointedly humiliating, aimed at gaining laughter. One of them asked, "How dare you tell me that I don't need to diet? I've spent decades of my life dieting and being miserable—how dare you suggest I didn't need to do it?" Anger is a normal response to being told that one's efforts, often span-ning one's whole adult life, have been meaningless.

The anger can be all encompassing—every article, every comment—becomes an attack not only on one's own body but on nonconforming bodies everywhere. How dare they? How dare anyone persist in believing these lies? Once we recognize injustice we see it every-where and we are furious. It's what we do with our fury that matters.

As a child I was fascinated by what the late-afternoon setting sun did to my shadow cast onto the sidewalk outside my home—my round shape would produce a shape taller and more slender. That is what I'm supposed to look like, I would think, even at seven or eight years old. That is what I shall look like when I am grown up. Evenings I would dance with my shadow on the sidewalk of my street, strolling, running, leaping in the air, to see how my future self—thinner, taller, more graceful in every way—would do these things. I would whisper my dreams to her, as though I could speak through time: you will wear jeans from the girls' department; you will be good at sports; you will be first picked for everything; people will never mistake you for a boy again.

In early 1994, the video for Queen Latifah's "U.N.I.T.Y." was in constant rotation on MTV. I was seventeen and my taste in music trended toward the intentionally and stubbornly obscure, but I still watched MTV. In the first verse, Latifah raps:

> . . . One day I was walking down the block
> I had my cutoff shorts on right 'cause it was crazy hot
> I walked past these dudes when they passed me
> One of 'em felt my booty, he was nasty

I turned around red, somebody was catching the wrath
Then the little one said, "Yeah me, bitch," and laughed
Since he was with his boys he tried to break fly
Huh, I punched him dead in his eye and said,
"Who you calling a bitch?"

These events are dramatically reenacted in the video, with Latifah—tall, thick, intimidating as hell in the best possible way—walking down a street in shorts when she is literally assaulted by a dude passing in the other direction with his friends. I saw this video for the first time on the tiny thirteen-inch TV in my old bedroom late at night, while I was waiting for *120 Minutes* to come on. I was rapt. At the time my draconian adherence to music snobbery prevented me from openly enjoying the song, but the video left a dramatic impression on me.

It wasn't so much that Latifah was all that big; I watch the video today and she seems pretty average. But at the time, she and I were close to the same size and I thought of myself as unfathomably massive, so much so that I had accepted the idea that nothing of note or merit would ever happen to me so long as I was fat—positive sexual attention from men included.

Fat women learn early that they should take male sexual attention wherever they can get it and to be damn grateful for it, because what self-respecting man would want to fuck a fat woman? Not only does this knowledge reinforce the idea that fat women do not deserve to be seen, but it also positions fat women as targets for men looking for an easy lay—she'll take what she can get, regardless of what she actually desires, and consider herself lucky. The idea of such a woman ever saying no is inconceivable; having actually been a woman saying no, I speak from experience. Men do not take it well when a woman they consider to be beneath their standards turns them down. Of course, this system is also oppressive of men. A dude who is specifically attracted to fatter women—and they do exist—is pathologized or called a fetishist, when nobody says the same about men who are specifically attracted to thinner women. Men are not enabled to be open about such an attraction unless they are willing to suffer the jibes of their friends, or maintain a constant politicized vigilance on the matter, and hey, men who do that exist as well.

But when I was seventeen I hadn't worked all this out yet, and seeing Latifah respond with such decisive and forceful resistance to the dude who grabs her was a revelation. It crystallized my nascent thinking that I should be allowed to refuse sexual attention when it was unwelcome. More than that, it gave me a better blueprint for standing up for myself. In this video and song, Latifah manages to speak her rage with intelligence, strength, and even humor, and when confronted with violence she is capable of responding in kind.

In the sixth grade, I had an admirer. I use the term with a healthy dose of irony, as his interest in me was limited to an apparent longing to put his hand inside my pants. He made frequent attempts each day—surreptitiously, silently, often during class, where we sat side-by-side in the back corner of the room. I presume he did it there because I was unlikely to make a scene in a room filled with our peers and a teacher. It was my fault he was doing it, of course. I was the one to feel ashamed. Yelling or otherwise reacting strongly to his gropes would mean I would either have to reveal my humiliating secret—that I was somehow unwittingly inviting this boy to grab at me—or keep it to myself and get in trouble for disrupting class for no good reason. So I said nothing. This is how boys, and later men, learn to target and prey on women—by exploiting female socialization to avoid making a spectacle of ourselves.

He was small for his age, with a curiously tall, curving forehead that gave the impression of a receding hairline, a strange thing to see on a twelve-year-old. His hands were likewise diminutive and uncomfortably hot. I could often sense his approach before he made contact with my knee or thigh. For several months, my means of warding him off was to rapidly shift position in my seat whenever he made an attempt. Being chastised by the teacher for fidgeting was better than the alternatives. One day when I'd had enough, I grabbed his hand and twisted as hard as I could, no longer caring if I got in trouble. It had to hurt, especially since I was markedly bigger and stronger than he, and though he flushed and grimaced he made no sound at all. And so I began to pinch him as fiercely as possible each time he tried to grope me. I'm sure the teacher thought we were playing or flirting, but the truth was I was in a near-constant state of terror and anxiety. Because I believed it was my fault, there was no one I could tell.

It all ended one day when I crushed his groping hand against a desk as I was standing to respond to an oral quiz, and something broke. It was an accident, or at least it looked like one, but then no one else knew how I had fantasized about the torture of the boy's appendages after months and months of stress and constant vigilance.

When Latifah appeared on my television years later preaching indignantly, "I punched him dead in his eye," it was as though by hearing this validation my urge of violent resistance was sated. I didn't need to react with force anymore, because it was enough to know that I could.

The idea of fatness as something other than an embarrassment or a temporary ailment came to me after encountering Susan Stinson's novel, *Fat Girl Dances with Rocks*, which I read slowly, standing up in the late, lamented Tower Records on Newbury Street, when I was nineteen years old. I spotted the book while browsing, and I paused because I had seen it mentioned in *Sassy* magazine when I was in high school. I told myself that I wasn't going to buy it because I was a student and dollars were scarce, but the truth was that I wasn't going to buy it because it had the word "fat" on the cover, and bringing such a book to the register would be like allying myself with that word. Instead, I went back to Tower Records daily, after class, and stole the book, page by page, word by word, by reading it in the store. The unhappy ending to this story came when someone bought it—or else it was moved or otherwise lost—and I felt deep regret that I didn't have a copy to finish.

A few years later I mustered the courage to buy another fat-titled book—there weren't many in the late 1990s—from the fledgling website amazon.com. It was, unsurprisingly, Marilyn Wann's seminal *Fat!So?*, and the rest is history.

I've been doing fat—living it, performing it, questioning it, and deconstructing it—in one way or another since then. I burned through *Fat!So?* in a single evening and began to memorize the statistics and arguments it contained, as tools, weapons even, to validate my continued existence. I'd had a lifetime of hating my body, for failing to be thin though I had worked harder for that goal than I'd thought possible. Wanting something to be real does not make it real, no matter how intensely you throw your want at it.

Occasionally, I'll still hear the voice asking, *you complain so much about the unfairness with which fat people are treated; why not just lose weight?* Even if assimilation is possible—and it very often is not—problems are not solved by assimilation. I am not confronting simply personal problems. I am defying and opposing all the social systems that value some appearance-based characteristics over others, and which contribute to a culture in which people who fail to comply—or who overtly resist—are punished. Everyone deserves respect and justice no matter what they look like. You are not required to be awesome in your fatness. I do not need you to be awesome in your fatness in order for me to feel justified in being awesome in my own. You *can* be awesome in your fatness, if you want, or you can choose another way to be. I will continue on with my own life in my own body no matter what you decide. I just want you to know that *awesomeness is possible*. As I've said before, your body is not a tragedy. It is the only one you get, no matter how it may challenge, confound, frustrate, or thrill you, and fighting your body isn't worth the hurt and the divide.

The overwhelming majority of fat people who have been on television in recent years have been featured on one unfortunately titled show, *The Biggest Loser*, a reality show with a simple premise: contestants compete to lose weight. The series came on air in the US in 2004, and has spawned over twenty international variations—proving that there is a huge market for the public humiliation of fat people pretty much anywhere you go—as well as multitudes of diet books, DVDs, a video game, and even two *Biggest Loser* "resorts," where paying customers can get a piece of the reality-TV action.

The show is not simply a weight-loss competition; it is a weight-loss-by-any-means-necessary competition. It demands that its participants lose dangerous amounts of weight very quickly, often with little regard for their health or even their survival. Trainers and medical professionals who are not generally critical of weight loss have expressed concerns about the show, and a handful of former contestants have spoken out on the lengths to which they went to have the lowest weekly weigh-in possible, including intentionally dehydrating themselves. Many have regained the weight they lost.

Though *The Biggest Loser* has multiple trainers, the best known one is Jillian Michaels. Michaels yells, a lot. She makes violent threats against her charges when they dare complain that the sudden imposition of six to seven hours of intense exercise on a (usually) sedentary body is too much, in one case screaming at a man, "The only way you're coming off this damn treadmill is if you die on it." She dehumanizes her *Biggest Loser* clients with vicious name-calling. She seems to think the brains of fat people have been compromised such that they can only respond to repetitive screaming. Her abuse is calculated to break her clients down until they weep, and even then she doesn't let up. She is often unpredictable, with a brutal and quick temper, and is apathetic toward (if not gratified by) her clients' physical and emotional discomfort. There are even elements of codependency—only when the fat people in question behave as instructed does her mood change and they may receive some warm encouragement or support, which is meted out in doses small enough to keep them craving more. Before any of this happens, her trainees must first be convinced that *they cannot possibly survive without her*, that their lives prior have been worthless, their bodies but hollow shells—or, in this case, shells filled with soulless fat.

Michaels' behavior in any other context would be abhorrent, if not considered outright abusive. But because she directs it only at fat people, it is allegedly for their own good and millions of people love it. They say, "Yeah! That's what these fat people need! They need to be abused!" And even some fat people love it. They say, "Yeah! That's what I need! I need a stranger to scream hurtful things at me while I exercise! Because she *cares*!" The reality is that many fat people believe they deserve humiliation and disrespect, that their grotesque fat has to be beaten out of them, emotionally or otherwise. That their evil has to be exorcised. That they and their bodies are not entitled to care and dignity, only punishment and pain.

Self-respect and self-esteem are not acquired automatically along with a slimmed-down body. How you do or do not value yourself is something that you will carry throughout the bodily changes that will inevitably take place in your lifetime. If you love yourself unconditionally—as you should, even if no one else does—then fatter or thinner, you are at home in your body. You neither want nor need abusive outsiders to instruct you on how to survive. This model of weight-loss-by-abuse is irresponsible, designed to produce good television more than to encourage healthier lifestyles. Our culture's hatred of fat bodies is enabled and reinforced; if Michaels is allowed to berate fat people under the auspices of doing them a favor, then certainly others are free to openly mock the next fat woman they see. Even if she's with her family. Even if she seems to be having a good time. How *dare* she?

There was a boy in middle school whose name escaped my memory long ago, though I can still see his face in my mind's eye and I can recall his voice with absolute clarity. He wasn't an unattractive boy, but he was the kind of boy that girls of that age don't much look at—tall and gangly with a notable lack of charm and self-assurance. Sometimes I try to imagine him today, twenty-something years on. Does he have a family, possibly a child rapidly approaching the age we were then? Did his life turn out the way he'd hoped? Is he happy?

We had a few classes together: science, math, and my favorite, journalism, which was really just a creative writing credit with a special designation. He must have known my name. The middle school I attended was not small, with over eight hundred kids in my graduating class, but we always knew the names of our most immediate peers. Nonetheless, at some point in our shared middle school lives he took to calling me "Obese."

I don't mean he called me obese as in, "Wow, girl, you are obese!" I'd heard that many times, before and after this boy's appearance in my world. I had been called obese and fat and the names of blubbery members of the animal kingdom as well. I'd also been called ugly, scary, stupid, disgusting, and many others of children's favorite adjectives for those who stand apart—by accident or by design—in some way.

But that's not what I mean when I say he called me obese. I mean he called me Obese, as though it was my name. He did it loudly, too, with a cheery, booming cadence that emphasized the second syllable: Oh-*bese*! Like a carnival barker, like a town crier. Oh-*bese*! *Come gawk at the fattest girl in the class, the fattest girl in the whole world, larger than you can imagine!*

"Fat" was not a word I used in those days. It was a word I avoided, a word I feared. I was not fat; *I was dieting.* I believed the popular lie that my weight was but a casing for my real inner self, which was thin. One day I would cast off my fatness like an overcoat and become my true thin body. Calling oneself fat was akin to admitting one was doomed forever. There is a finality to it, a sound of settling earth, an abandonment of hope, a giving up on the successful transformation, a decisive sadness, a sacrifice of the dream. My size was purely temporary, an accident, I told myself, of my parents' divorce when I was six.

Something had happened to derail my natural thin development. I once overheard my father, in whose custody I remained following my parents' divorce, say he thought perhaps my size was his fault, that in the absence of a governing influence, he fed me too much, without my mother around to mete out appropriate portions. I clung to the story for years because it gave me a reason. It explained things. I can honestly say I was never angry at my father, nor did I blame him—I was simply relieved to know why it had happened and that it was not owing to any moral failure on my part.

Whether the boy knew my name or not is probably irrelevant, though the question lingers in my mind still. Was I even a person to him? I can't remember the voice of my grandfather who passed away when I was seventeen, or my best friend from that middle school era, but I remember *his* voice and the way he said Oh-*bese*! to me, over and over, every day. It echoes in my mind like an audible scar. He said it when people were around, in crowded classrooms and the cafeteria. He said it when I was the only one present, if he caught me in the hallway or walking out to the buses at the end of the day. Once in that journalism class, he bellowed it multiple times in rapid succession as I tried to take my seat and I thought *shut up shut up shut up shutupshut-upshutpSHUTUP* hoping to will him into silence so that none of my other classmates would pick up on his taunt and start calling me by that name as well. When the bell rang, the teacher, whom I idolized, shut him down with a quiet "That's enough." Why didn't she say more? Did she think I was an obese monster too, that my real name wasn't even worth speaking? Did everyone?

I have a photograph of myself from the day I graduated the eighth grade. I am standing at the end of the sun-dappled front walk of the peach-painted stucco house in South Florida. I am wearing a cream-colored, midcalf-length dress, gathered at the waist, with a matching brocade jacket. The jacket has trim made of plastic "pearls" edging the open front and the sleeve openings, which digs into the skin of my upper arms, just a bit, enough to be irritating. My hair is huge, teased and sprayed into a nearly spherical halo of honey-tinged curls. I am wearing dyed-to-match, kitten-heeled satin pumps. I was fourteen then, and I look remarkably similar to how I look today, not because I have aged well, but because in the picture I look at least a decade older than I was. The dress came from an upscale plus-size store in the mall. My mother took me there once our initial expeditions in search of a formal dress revealed to us both that I could no longer shop in straight-size stores. I was simply too big.

We didn't call them plus sizes then. I knew them as "women's sizes," often carried by stores with "woman" somewhere in the name. Even at fourteen I found this confusing as it seemed to imply that smaller sizes were less woman-y, and this flew in the face of what I understood about how my fat made my peers see me as less legitimately female—a girl in name only. The fat ones were certainly not the girls who got asked to school dances. The fat ones were an abomination of "normal" girlhood, and yet here the clothes were made for *women*. It made no sense.

It was, after all, a euphemism: women's sizes were no more womanly, nor were the women who wore them. It was—and is—simply less offensive to give those clothes an innocuous yet purposeful title, be it "woman" or "plus," to set them apart. It is also a subliminal compliment: *you're still a woman!* the store's name might seem to suggest. *Pay a lot of money for a poorly made garment from us, since we told you that!* Because, one might argue, who would shop in a store that openly calls its customers fat?

So my mom and I wound up at this upscale plus-size boutique in search of an appropriate dress. I felt no embarrassment or shame in being there; indeed, I remember only feeling relief that a store existed where I could fit into everything it carried, matronly though the options were, having spent so many years squeezing myself into the too-small biggest sizes at Lerner's and Express and The Limited. The salesladies fawned over me—I doubt they had many customers under the age of forty—and eventually I left with the dress described above.

Today my mom says, "I know you like to poke fun at yourself, but you really did look gorgeous in that dress."

I explain, "It wasn't that I think I looked bad. It's that I looked totally different from all the other fourteen-year-olds I was graduating with." My peers wore flimsy dresses from juniors shops in the mall, cheap synthetic stuff that likely cost one third what we paid, and yet I would have been just as happy to fit in with them at the time.

Now when I took at pictures of my middle school self, I don't see a fat girl. I see a round face; I see a noncurvy figure, as I have never been small waisted or large bosomed or traditionally "womanly" in shape at any point in my life. I see a girl who was probably a bit taller and wider than some of her classmates, but who was not really different to any dramatic degree. I certainly don't see the gargantuan freak of nature I believed I was then, which was probably at least slightly related to the fact that there was a kid who called me Obese as though it was my name.

Today I can look back at my eighth grade picture and think, *Wow, I really wasn't all that fat.* But the sharper truth is that even at the time, telling me I wasn't fat wouldn't have helped. Telling me I wasn't fat would have done nothing to quell my insecurities, my gutter-level self-esteem, my passionate body hatred. Telling me I wasn't fat, even if you told me every day, wouldn't have changed a thing about my self-image. I knew I was fat, and the reality of it was irrelevant. I knew it with all the certainty of my burgeoning adolescence.

What would have been helpful? It would have been helpful to hear that I deserved not to be bullied or taunted, regardless of my size. It would have been helpful to hear that my being fat was a not reason to hate myself, starve myself, hurt myself, or punish my body for failing to conform to the images in my head or in the magazines I read. It would have been helpful to hear that being fat was not the end of my world, that it did not mean nobody would ever love me or want to be my friend. It would have been helpful to hear that, yes, even if you are obese, you still deserve a basic modicum of dignity and respect. These are the things that would have helped; these are the things that may have saved me years of damage that took additional years to repair. What was singularly unhelpful was being told I wasn't fat in the first place, since that assertion did nothing to dismantle the idea that fat people richly deserve their ill treatment. Being identified as "not fat" meant the fear of becoming fat (or fatter) was allowed to remain solidly intact.

I n February of 2010, First Lady Michelle Obama announced a public health campaign, the kind of seemingly innocuous, apolitical effort that first ladies have made for a few administrations now. Michelle Obama's campaign was called Let's Move and it focused on eliminating childhood obesity within one generation.

On the surface, it didn't seem like a bad idea. Sure, it's unfortunate that the campaign had to be pegged with the keywords "childhood obesity" to get attention, but the effort's stated intentions were reasonable. It promised to improve school lunch options and to provide better funding for physical education. It argued in favor of better access to nutrition information and higher quality foods for families. It is difficult to argue with such good intentions.

But at some point, things began to go wrong with the campaign.

For one thing, the language of the goal of Let's Move was troubling in itself: to "eliminate" or "eradicate" childhood obesity. While it may sound wonderfully optimistic, this goal is impossible. Fat children have existed throughout history and will continue to dangle from one end of the bell curve no matter what we do to them, institutionally, culturally, or socially. They cannot be eradicated. But the very suggestion that they ought to be, like an infestation, is troubling, as it positions fat children as objects both undesirable and disposable. I am not arguing that this is intentional, given that a thoughtful adult can see the subtle distinction between eliminating obesity in children and eliminating individual fat kids. But children cannot. And children are as likely to hear about this campaign as anyone.

Far-reaching public health campaigns like Let's Move obviously have the power to shape discourse, so it is important to think about the language we use to implement them. More than that, we must also consider how we position campaigns in the broader cultural exchange and the possible ramifications. In March of 2011, Michelle Obama delivered remarks to the National League of Cities Conference in Washington, DC. The National League of Cities is a nongovernmental organization that connects municipal leadership nationwide. Obama chose to discuss childhood obesity at this meeting. Her full speech can be read on whitehouse.gov, the official White House website. But I'd like to zero in on one point she makes, as it is a point being echoed by much of the media in their hysteria about obesity-as-crisis:

> [This is] an issue that can drastically alter the economic landscape of our cities and towns for generations to come. And I am obviously talking about the epidemic of childhood obesity. . . .
>
> You all know better than anyone that childhood obesity is already affecting your communities. It's already weighing down your budgets. It's already hampering economic growth.

Stunningly, it sounds as though Michelle Obama is blaming fat children, at least in part, for slow economic growth and high unemployment in the recession. She is not alone in this assessment, as the news media has been beating the same drum for awhile. Obama goes on to explain that the continued existence of these fat kids is putting their parents out of work by driving away new businesses from "unhealthy" towns. She also talks about how they are negatively affecting the military readiness of the United States, ostensibly because some fat kids grow up to be fat adults who don't make useful soldiers. Frankly I am surprised that Obama does not also manage to pin rising oil prices, urban poverty, and earthquakes on fat kids too, but I suppose there are limits.

Part of the trouble here is the way we define—or don't define—obesity. If obesity implies illness, then Obama's comments are easier to swallow. The problem is, unlike cancer or heart disease, obesity is not always a source of sickness. In January of 2010, Dr. Regina Benjamin, the US Surgeon General, posted a video on the Department of Health and Human Services' official YouTube channel in which she acknowledges the concern of obesity rates, but also says: "The good news is, we can be healthy and fit at any size or any weight. As America's family doctor, I want to change the national conversation from a negative one about obesity and illness, to a positive conversation about being healthy and being fit."

It's not surprising that we have heard little of this position since. Positive conversations do not scare people, nor do they place blame on groups of individuals for culture-wide problems. The concept of the scapegoat is mostly known as a biblical reference, described in Leviticus, home to some of the Bible's greatest hits so far as grotesqueries are concerned. It is in Leviticus, of course, that we get the alleged admonitions against homosexuality, eating shellfish, and planting two different seeds in the same field. As Leviticus tells it, in order to make a scapegoat, you take a couple of goats and draw lots against them. The winning goat gets sacrificed (how this is a win, I don't know). The loser goat is symbolically heaped with the sins of the community and sent off into the wilderness, dragging the invisible pile of sin with it, possibly much to the relief of the goat who may now wander the forest eating rocks or doing whatever it is that free goats do. The idea behind this ritual is that the loser goat somehow absorbs all the bad that has been done in the community, and when it leaves, it takes the evil with it.

The ancient Greeks had a similar practice. They selected a *pharmakos*—usually someone disabled, ugly, or some other social outcast—and placed the blame for troubled times upon him or her. The *pharmakos* would then be removed from the community as a means of correcting the issue at hand, such as a famine or a flood. The Greek version is even more gruesome than the biblical one, as in their ritual the *pharmakos* was not merely driven into the wilderness but often beaten or stoned to death. Then as now, people who are not attractive are disposable, indeed barely people at all, and serve as a convenient target on which to blame issues far beyond their control, because who will stand up for the right of the ugly or the disabled to survive?

The central problem with Let's Move and campaigns like it, which place an overwhelming emphasis on fat children in particular, is that they create a space in which scapegoating these children (and adults) seems logical and acceptable. It puts an official stamp on the existing cultural hatred of fatness and makes it seem legitimate. It implies that one of the most important things in a child's life should be the size and shape of his or her body. And what of the kids who cannot lose weight? These children, half-starved on diets, possibly surgically altered, routinely bullied, their parents openly embarrassed by them, their peers unwilling to accept them, must know that their continued existence is unacceptable. They must be told! Of course, the simplest route to this end is to blame them for sabotaging something that is a near-universal problem, something that concerns us all, something like the economy. We, with Michelle Obama's help, will *eradicate you.*

Fat kids are not loser goats. Fat kids need support, reassurance, and encouragement, like all kids, but maybe even a little bit more. Fat kids are kids to whom adults must demonstrate a specific sensitivity and thoughtfulness to counteract the hate and bullying that even kindergarten-age children already know they are culturally entitled to heap on their fat peers. Fat kids need advocacy that does not single them out from their thinner counterparts but treats them equally.

All kids benefit from the assistance of adults and public health initiatives to become more active, eat a wide variety of healthy foods, and learn to know their bodies and their abilities. Not all thin kids are inherently healthy, and inadequate nutrition can take a serious toll even on "normal"-looking children. With exercise and improved diet, sure, some fat kids are likely to stop being fat—and some aren't. But this is not the point. The point is to improve the overall health and fitness of *all* kids, and for this to happen these children must be allowed to thrive in an environment that does not shame them and their bodies, but instead teaches them that their bodies are awesome machines and that every one is different, sometimes in ways that are dramatic and sometimes in ways that are subtle.

Fat kids deserve love and respect. They deserve to be given room to be their best selves. But by blaming fat children for the ills of a nation and thereby reinforcing an already powerful cultural bias against them, Michelle Obama is rapidly becoming the biggest bully of them all, despite her good intentions. Her work on this issue cannot possibly succeed in improving children's health when so much of it rests on engendering prejudice and shame. Let's Move does not have to focus on the elimination of fat children; it can focus on improving the education and health of kids of all sizes, and of their parents too. When children have poor access to healthy food options and nowhere safe to be active, it is not only the fat kids who suffer. All children living in such circumstances—subsisting in food deserts, poverty, underfunded schools, neighborhoods without open spaces to play in—whether they are fat or thin, are at risk. The long-term consequences of poor nutrition not only cost money when they happen to make a kid fat. This focus on childhood obesity is simply unnecessary when these issues affect every child at every size.

I did not see that boy again, the Oh-*bese*! boy, after I went to high school, and for many years I had forgotten about him altogether. It was only later, hearing myself referred to as obese again by the ubiquitous pack of teenagers shouting from a moving car, that I remembered him. By that point I had resisted terms like "overweight" and "obese" in favor of "fat" for altogether different reasons. Those terms turn fat bodies into a pathology, an illness, a disease to be cured, and I did not take kindly to having my body referred to in this way.

"Overweight" bears up the notion that body size is a uniform thing, that there is a particular range of weights for every given height within which one is either "under" or "over." Overweight carries with it a distinct sense of temporariness: this is not my actual weight, I am "over" that at present. When we are overweight, we are comparing ourselves to a certain standard. Whether that standard is determined for us by a line on a chart, or whether we decide where our overweight begins, the point is that this body is abnormal at this time, but it may not always be so. Overweight suggests one is undergoing a bodily shift, a problem to be solved.

"Obese," on the other hand, implies affliction and disease. Obese is not a simple descriptor like "tall," or "wearing a hat." It is medical, technical, and value-laden: it is not an insult so much as a dire assessment. Obesity is routinely framed in discourse as not only a disease but an *epidemic*, a word strongly associated with the rampant threat of illness, and worse, contagion, requiring constant vigilance. Obesity will get you, as it has gotten so many of us, so watch out for it.

Neither "overweight" nor "obese" have any real place outside of their natural habitat of medical conversations, and yet they are used routinely in the vernacular, particularly by the media. Why? Because these words are scary, and they make people worry and thereby pay attention. On a culture-wide level, a population that is living under constant threat of illness is a tractable one, and there are financial and social benefits to be reaped by using language to subtly promote a terror of obesity. How many people are obese according to the numbers and don't even know it? This is a prospective horror all its own. But ultimately obese is just a word, and a word cannot make you sick, nor can it kill you, although it can make you feel bad about yourself if you let it.

We have a great many other words we use when we are not comfortable using the word fat, which is almost all of the time. I'm not fond of euphemisms. Even as a fat child I did not often use the friendlier terms intended to soften the blow: chubby, chunky, pudgy, plump, fluffy (yes, fluffy, as though one's body is the result of an overly generous application of fabric softener). I didn't use the word "fat" either, owing to its power as the worst insult of all, and instead I relied on vague and neutral terms like "big" and "bigger."

A euphemism's purpose is to sidestep possible unpleasant associations with more straightforward language, or to avoid coming across as rude. Of course, if a euphemism works, it still gets the point across, it just uses a different word to do it. Calling a fat person fluffy does not render them any less fat, but it does bypass any negative connotations the person may have with "fat" as a word. Fat people are gross, as everyone knows; euphemistically described people are not like those gross fat people, even if their bodies are similar.

"Plus size" comes from the sizing distinction made by clothing manufacturers and retailers, a group that is probably not the best resource for determining how to describe our bodies, but given the inclination of women to shape themselves to fit their clothes and not the other way around, it is an unsurprising one.

Indeed, plus size and fat are distinct concepts, but not exclusive. Fat people are often plus size by default, but not all plus-size people are fat. Plus size is a matter of accessibility; fat is a matter of substance. The difference is rather one of personal appreciation and semantics. Plus size, by its connection to clothing, also suggests a connection with plus-size models, who are generally fat only by the strictest standards of the fashion industry, and look altogether normal by most cultural standards. (Indeed, plus-size modeling starts at a size ten, which is not a plus size by any definition.) The implication of "plus size" as a euphemism is *you're not fat, you just wear a bigger size in clothing.*

"Curvy" is another popular euphemism for fatness, one that is similarly deployed as code for a few distinguishing characteristics that separate the body in question from the more negative connotations of "fat." Primarily, curvy implies proportional, usually a standard hourglass figure, but scaled up. It's an attractive body that mostly looks like the idealized thinner version—the distinct waist, the wider hips, the bust line in balance with both—but . . . thicker. The problem here is that there are millions of women who do not fit that description, and who are thus led down the garden path to believing that their salvation lies in either Machiavellian attempts to remake their shapes (through surgery, deprivation, or abuse) or, if and when they meet with failure, resenting or even hating their natural bodies. Curvy is not helpful when there are fat women without narrow waists; there are slender women who lack rounded hips; there are women of all sizes whose breasts fail to conform to a size aesthetically in step with the rest of their bodies. Our world is riddled with the struggles of women trying to pull themselves from the self-loathing pit while impossible beauty standards repeatedly push them back down again. Curvy, in an attempt to be positive, still privileges certain acceptably feminine shapes at the expense of others, and for those of us who ain't curvy—I count myself among this group—it can be far more alienating and patronizing than fat ever is. Good intentions be damned, curvy still creates an arbitrary standard of acceptability, albeit one that is *slightly larger* than the current one.

In recent years, "real" has gained traction as a popular euphemism, well-intentioned though ultimately misguided. The notion that fat women—or at least plus-size women—are real women is even underscored by ubiquitous polyester-horror outlet Lane Bryant, which frequently uses the term in its marketing materials. Real sets up a handy dualism in which women who are not thin are pitted against women who are in a battle to exist. The message is that models are not real (except they are) and women who are normally very slender are not real either; the challenge to their reality is not simply an attack on their right to be, but on their womanhood in particular. Real women have curves. Men prefer real women. Real is an apt term to employ for a group of women who feel erased by culture, because they cannot see their bodies represented in the media onslaught that bears down on us every day. Real is also an interesting detour from diet ideology that promises to reveal one's true slender body hiding under all that fat. By calling non-skinny bodies real, we are arguing in favor of our bodies' authenticity even in our fatter states.

The problem with real is that it identifies other bodies as fake, and if real is positive, then fake must be negative. The bodies in opposition to this reality are bodies that are thin, bodies that are overly perfect, bodies that have undergone plastic surgery. Fake bodies are hypothetically without the flaws that would make them real, and yet I'm sure if you talked to any fake-body-having-woman she would have as many issues with her appearance as anyone else. Fake bodies are also by extension unnatural, and our collective cultural revulsion against the unnatural is deeply entrenched. Very slender women who despise their bodies may even be pitied for their inability to gain flesh in their hips and breasts; their ability to be "natural" has been thwarted, no matter how much they eat.

Thus, many of the words we use to circumlocute fat can be as damaging as fat would be, albeit their damage is more cultural and less individual. And our negative connotations with fat are unsurprising. In the dominant discourse, fat is a word treated with the reverence some hold for ethnic slurs. It is not a word to be used lightly, and when it is deployed, the intention is clear: fat transmits not only an observation of the state of one's physical body, but bears more menacing implications for their character, their habits, and the condition of their immortal soul.

Fat is routinely paired with gender-specific insults like slut, bitch, and whore. A fat slut is not merely a sexually promiscuous woman, but a sexually promiscuous woman with whom no decent man would want to have sex. A fat slut is a woman whose sexuality is itself wrong and offensive, because fatness precludes sexual attractiveness. A fat slut is a problem because if a woman is mostly good for sex, and she dares be fat, she has no purpose; her usefulness is eclipsed by her failure to be sexually appealing, or even sexually accessible in a literal, physical way. The bodies of fat sluts are recognized as a barrier to their penetration, and that simply won't do. If she wants it, she must not make it so difficult for a man to give it to her. Fat, in this context, is shorthand for ugly, but there is more to it than that. Fat also represents a perceived lack of control, an appetite—for food or sex—that is unmanaged and unseemly. A fat slut simply devours, with no regard for herself or anyone else; she is culturally despicable as a figure who consumes resources without producing anything of value. She is barely a woman; she is the ruination of women.

Beyond its use as a gendered insult, fat is the tiny word on which the guilt of a culture rests. Try telling someone you are pro-fat, in favor of fatness, a person who advocates for fattery on an epic scale. See how they react. Expressing a pro-fat position is on a par with extolling the joys of kicking defenseless puppies or selling drugs to schoolchildren. This reaction is typical even in fat-acceptance circles. We are not supposed to be pushing for everyone to be fat, you see, we are merely asking for our own individual fatness to be accepted.

B ack in November of 2008, I wrote something online in which I used the phrase "death fat" as a counter-euphemism for "morbidly obese."

Though "morbidly" has since been phased out of the medical parlance—in favor of class II and class III obesities, which are far less hysterically ominous—its original use seemed to imply that fat people of a certain size, myself included, were so very fat that they were in danger of imminent death-by-obesity.

I couldn't have predicted how people would connect with the idea—and how many of them would come to use the term to describe themselves, as I did. Death fat is funny. It mocks the concept of morbid obesity as determined by the BMI scale, which fails to consider the overall health of the individual in question, and damns them as walking corpses based exclusively on their poundage. Death fat points out that morbid obesity is an absurdly overwrought turn of phrase, given the simple reality that not everyone who falls under this category is in imminent danger—or even long-term danger—of a fat-related demise.

The humor in death fat is critical. Laughter relieves stress. For example, the stress of living as a fat person who is told routinely—by an individual and/or by cultural discourse as a whole—that they are morally suspect, intellectually inferior, physically disgusting, and/or ultimately doomed to die (unlike, uh, everyone else). Ultimately, I employ death fat as a means of gently poking fun at strangers who would get all wrought up over their professed concerns about my health.

Health is both private and subjective. My health is none of your business. Your health is none of mine. The health of the barista who hands you your coffee in the morning? None of your business. The health of your postal carrier? None of your business. The health of a particular film star or professional athlete? None of your business. The health of a fat stranger walking down the street in front of you? None of your business.

If our culture is going to wield the threat of death as a motivational factor to assimilate, I am going to smile patiently and nod and admit, yes, it's true, someday I'm going to die. But it won't be after spending my whole life miserably chasing a body I'm not meant to have. It won't be after spending my whole life hating my body and doubting myself. And in the end it's not something you need to worry about either. Don't let your own life pass you by because you're trying to tell me how to live mine.

Learning to say the word fat may be one of the most difficult points on your journey. It was for me. Giving up on dieting—that was easy. It had never worked anyway, and even someone as stubborn as myself will eventually stop beating her head against a brick wall once she realizes that the brick wall is unchanged while my head has suffered all the damage. The loathing of my body, that was a bit harder, but overcoming that was a similarly organic process of assessing any self-imposed ruin and accepting that this was the body I got to live in and no amount of hatred was going to get me a different one. But saying the word? Saying the word was a bridge I had to build board-by-board and nail-by-nail until I got to the other side.

Fat is a word with power, a word with a social investment, like a pyramid of assumption, expectation, and stereotype balanced upside down on its point. It is by fearing this word and letting its connotations be dictated to us that we perpetuate its use as an insult and a weapon. I make a habit of rephrasing euphemistic speech in the most straightforward language possible, with fat at the center: I am not morbidly obese, I am death fat. It isn't an obesity epidemic: it is a fat rampage.

Fat.

Say it out loud. It's a good word. Sharp, decisive, monosyllabic—it strikes at the eardrum like an explosion, like gunfire, an assault. Fat is a beginning and an end all in one quick motion. Be aware of every letter and skip none. Feel the F's aggressive vibrations on your lower lip, the bright sting of the short A, the crisp conclusion of the T.

Once my partner asked me why I say the word fat as I do. "How do I say it?" I asked. He couldn't explain. He was unsure if it was the pronunciation or the emphasis or the way I'd crash the word out into conversation, into public spaces, where it shatters all comfort and gentility and leaves an atonal screech hanging in the suddenly silent air, like a needle coming off a record.

How do I say it? I speak fat like a language, like a reminder, like a flag of conquest. I wield it like a weapon, like a narrow spear driven into soft spaces between armored plates, so that people listen with my point pricking in their sides. How do I say it? I spit the word with eagerness and joy, eyes alight with the anticipation of how those who hear will react. I see the reactions of the folk who are unaccustomed to the word: they jump as if electrically shocked, they startle, and whatever they were thinking of is suddenly wiped from their minds—*did she just call herself fat?*

I see the reactions of the folk who use the word as I do, the cackling glee with our shared dialect, our secret password that is a secret to no one who can observe our bodies. We smile and laugh and elbow one another with shared delight. We are rebels, criminals, we are coming for your sons and daughters, and you cannot use that word against us anymore. No, it is our word now, whether it rests in your mouths or in ours.

This word fat is a souvenir, thrust from my throat and the space between my lungs with all the emphasis and force with which it is flung at me by strangers as an insult. I have earned it. It belongs to me now. You'll never take it back.

We live in a culture and economy that is driven by consumption, yet our relationship with our consuming behaviors is conflicted. We define ourselves, in part, by the things we consume, yet we also feel guilt for consuming too much. The items we buy, the stuff we collect, the clothing we wear, the television shows we watch, the books and magazines we read—these things carry identifying characteristics that often attract us as much as the content of the artifacts themselves. Even when we choose to consume things that are label-free, or socially conscious, that itself is a signal of who we are.

Since we derive so much from our consumption, it is hardly surprising that fat bodies, and thereby fat people, would come to represent the social outcast, the uncontrolled appetite, the selfish, the greedy, the slovenly. The myth of the overeating, overconsuming, constantly expanding fatass persists because of this association, because bodies are also commodified and consumed. We consume images of impossibly beautiful bodies every day, and we learn to relate to all bodies as consumable objects. You can buy the tits you always wanted, a younger face, a slimmer ass. You can buy it all from plastic surgeons or from the manufacturers of physics-defying undergarments or from Jenny Craig or the author of the fad-diet book du jour. The fat body is itself consumed by diets, surgery, "willpower," and once it has been swallowed, digested, and discarded, those who accomplish this feat of consumption are heralded as heroes of restraint, redeemed sinners, the hope of a nation. Their stories go on to be consumed by others who hope to replicate their success and the cycle goes on and on. There are numerous celebrities and other public figures whose fame rests as much on their ability to lose and gain weight as their ability to entertain or inform. I could give you names, but by the time you read these words, many of them may be fat again. Or thin again. Or fat again, thin again, fat again.

We can't be allowed to have fat bodies, you understand, because the fat body represents guilt, a lack of self-control, and, on a class-based note, a gauche display of abundance. Fat bodies are unseemly because they demonstrate that we have too much, here in the US in particular. Fast food is cheap and plentiful with ever-increasing portions and "value" meals that rapidly become inedible unless they are consumed immediately. Excellent produce and other whole foods are expensive and often impractical when we can get processed foods in greater volume for less money. We blame statistics that tell us that obesity is dispro-portionately common among poor folks who are too dumb to eat properly and exercise. *What they need is education!* No. What they need is access, time, and maybe a little more institutionalized support. But that is unlikely to happen because fat bodies must continue to exist as a cautionary tale, and who better to leave that job to than the poor? They're used to doing the tasks no one else wants.

I weigh something in the neighborhood of three hundred pounds.

What is the exact number? I have no idea. Truth is, I haven't been on a scale for at least three years, and the time before that was many more years still. My relationship with scales can most charitably be described as tense, and more accurately as harrow-ing. Unless a medical provider can give me a specific reason for needing to know more about my fatness than can be told simply by looking at me, I do not get on the scale at the doctor's office, and I certainly don't get on a scale anywhere else. At one time, it was a fear of the number that kept me back, but now it is more a desire to avoid the psychological effects of The Scale Experience, an event that was the source of incredible anxiety and self-loathing for the better part of my childhood and adolescence. I can keep an awareness of my size via body measurements, which do not hold the same emotional import. The scale is a traumatic place, a place I prefer not to go.

Hanne Blank, the amazing writer, historian, and badass queer fat lady who I am lucky to call a friend, was the first person whom I heard say it was okay to refuse the scale at the doctor's office. Hanne calls it "post-traumatic scale disorder," by which she explains the tendency to have disordered thinking as a result of being summed up as a number—a number that is considered abnormal. If our weight has been consistent, one might argue that there is nothing diagnostic that the scale will reveal, and therefore the traumatic experience of stepping on it is entirely unnecessary. It has certainly been my experience that medical professionals can tell that I am fat simply by looking at me.

At the Fat Girl Flea Market in New York, an annual fundraiser and clothing sale, a sea of fat bodies, most of them hot and sweating, shoulder to fat shoulder, try on clothing together. Why bother using the changing area? We're all fat here. Each body is unique, like a fingerprint of flesh, some shaped in ways familiar and some in ways utterly foreign. There is jostling and nudging; it isn't sexual, it's functional. This is one of very few spaces where you can touch someone with your fat flesh and not feel compelled to withdraw immediately, expecting revulsion from the person in receipt. When political fatties meet, we crush each other with hugs. There is relief in that exchange, in shared spatial understanding.

As it turns out, I am one of those annoying people who can eat whatever I want and not gain weight. This is as bewildering to me as it is to you.

Conventional wisdom is that a fat body is constantly expanding at an uncontrolled rate, given to explosion or collapse as a result of even small changes in diet. Fat people get fatter because they eat too much, which is why they are fat in the first place. Thin people, or simply "average" people, stay thin because they eat the correct amount, which is why they are not fat. But this logic does not apply to everyone.

My body size has not changed appreciably since 1999, when I moved from the walking-intensive city of Boston to the suburbs. I had been a student, operating on a student's income, and so city life was necessarily a spartan experience. My rent was astronomical, and even though I had a car, I rarely used it as parking was always a problem. The nearest MBTA stop was a good ten-minute walk from my apartment, and most of where I went—Boston University for school and Blockbuster Video for work—was best accessible via walking, and so I walked everywhere, everyday.

At this time I wasn't thin; I have never been thin. Not even close. At my very smallest, during a particularly dark and depressive period of my young adult life, I wore roughly a US women's size eighteen/twenty, but by 1999 I was wearing around a twenty-two/twenty-four. The move to the suburbs after college meant less walking, certainly, but at the same time I also started graduate school, which meant I was spending an obscene amount of each day sitting and reading or writing. And smoking cigarettes. I smoked lots and lots of cigarettes. (I've since quit. Kids, don't smoke.)

I don't actually know if any of this contributed to the weight I gained following the move. I was now cohabitating with the person I'd eventually marry, so maybe that was a factor. I changed birth control methods; maybe that was a factor. I quit smoking; maybe that was a factor. I was cooking actual meals for the first time in my life, rather than subsisting on ramen and macaroni and cheese; maybe that was a factor. Whatever the reason, I put on some degree of weight, not a huge amount, just enough that I shifted from wearing mostly one size to mostly another size, and some of my pants—I still wore pants, back then!—became too snug for comfort.

I put on about one dress size's worth of weight and then the weight gain stopped. I made some new clothes, donated the old pants, bought some cheap dresses at Marshalls. Problem solved.

Since then my weight has not changed at all. It does not matter if I eat or don't eat, or how much, or whether it's healthy foods or unhealthy foods. It doesn't even matter if I go to the gym regularly. For the past twenty years I have neither gained nor lost weight. I have dresses ten years old that fit the way they did when I bought them; if I'd had a proper wedding gown—the yardstick some women seem to use for their weight— it would fit me the same today as it did in 2003. (I do still own the outfit I wore to get married, and it fits.) I can't explain this in any way other than to say that different bodies are different and some bodies are just fat. No matter what we do to them, we are fat.

I f fatness is a medical problem, it makes logical sense that it should have a medical solution. Science (and quackery) has sought an obesity "cure" in pill form for as long as pills have existed. One study found that five million people used prescription weight loss drugs between 1996 and 1998 (interestingly, 25 percent of them were not overweight, suggesting a significant amount of abuse). However, the existence of these drugs, and the continuing research to find one that actually works, has cultural effects that reach beyond the individuals who use them. The existence and continued prescription of these drugs further underscores the ideology that fatness is an illness requiring medical intervention.

As of early 2011, there are only two prescription weight-loss drugs currently approved by the US Food and Drug Administration (FDA). They are orlistat (also known as Xenical, and available over the counter as Alli) and phentermine.

Orlistat is a "fat absorption inhibitor." That means it prevents dietary fats in the digestive tract from being broken down and consumed by your body. There is a huge downside because those fats still have to come out. For the handful of you unfamiliar with the horrors associated with this drug, please understand that the common side effects include "oily spotting in your undergarments; oily or fatty stools; orange or brown colored oil in your stool; gas with discharge, an oily discharge; loose stools, or an urgent need to go to the bathroom; inability to control bowel movements; an increased number of bowel movements . . . " I think my favorite of the above is "gas with discharge," which under any other circumstances would be called "shitting one's pants." And not only will this drug make you shit your pants, but the shit will be of an unusually disgusting quality even by shit's low standards. But don't worry! According to the drug's promotional materials, these "are actually signs that the medication is working properly."

Phentermine is best known as the "phen" in phen-fen, the popular off-label, diet-pill cocktail that caused permanent damage to some folks' heart valves, and at least one death many years ago. The plug got pulled on phen-fen when the "fen" half of the combination, fenfluramine, also known as Redux, took the bullet for the heart valve issues and was removed from the market in 1997. Phentermine, however, was determined to be an innocent bystander in those incidents, although its possible side effects include high blood pressure, tachycardia, and palpitations. Phentermine continues to be in use as a diet drug for its stimulant effects, filling the slot left by dangerous amphetamines used by millions of women in the 1950s and 1960s for weight loss.

In late 2010, a drug that had been approved by the FDA, marketed under the brand name Meridia, was pulled from shelves with much controversy. It was taken off the market on the basis of a study that found an increased risk of heart attacks, strokes, and related deaths among folks with pre-existing heart conditions. Meridia operated by altering brain chemistry and carried the banner of "appetite suppressant," though apparently it didn't work all that well. In clinical studies funded by the company that manufactured it, the average total weight loss while on the drug was five pounds. Of those who lost weight, 30 percent kept it off.

The rationale for removing Meridia was that its mediocre effectiveness was insufficient to justify the increased risk of heart attacks. Not everyone at the FDA agreed with the decision. In a particularly telling moment, one of the panelists who voted in favor of keeping Meridia on the market said in an article on *MSNBC*, "I think that just because we didn't measure the benefits scientifically doesn't mean they don't exist." Fortunately, science demands evidence and not faith in such matters.

How can it be that these drugs are continuing to be prescribed and used, when their usefulness is so limited, even according to the statistics put out by the manufacturers themselves? Weight loss is a business, and a profitable one at that. As of 2008, it has been estimated that the US spends between $33 and $55 billion on weight loss products and services annually. (For comparison, the entire US fashion industry had a revenue of about $14 billion in 2009.) The marketing and sale of weight loss drugs—like all diets, in fact—intentionally exploit our cultural investment in the power of the individual by encouraging folks to believe that even if the statistics are against you, you are going to be one of the lucky few to succeed where everyone else has failed. You are *special*, and all those other people are doing it wrong. You want it more than they did. And you deserve it.

In early 2011, a new diet drug came before the FDA advisory panel. The drug was called Contrave, and it basically didn't work. To be precise, it was considered only "modestly effective" by the panel. The FDA requirements for effectiveness in diet drug trials is that at least 35 percent of participants lose at least

5 percent of their body weight. For a three-hundred-pound person, that's fifteen pounds. To break it down further, the drug needs to produce a minimum loss of fifteen pounds in roughly one out of every three three-hundred-pound people who take it. Obviously, the loss would need to be even less for someone who weighs less to start with. That's it. Given that the panel was not "overly impressed" with the "modest weight loss" results of Contrave, it's probably safe to assume their numbers were not much above these minimum requirements.

Contrave also carried potential risks to cardiovascular health similar to those posed by Meridia, yet the panel recommended Contrave be approved. Why? According to panel chairman Abraham Thomas, head of endocrinology at Henry Ford Hospital in Detroit, quoted in *Reuters*, "My concern is . . . we will potentially kill development of these medications, and [obesity] is the most serious disease that the United States is facing." The panel did not recommend the drug be approved because it actually works, but to encourage the research and development of other weight-loss drugs.

If the FDA continues to reject weight-loss drugs, then companies will cease spending money to research them because drug companies are in business to make money, and there's no money to be made from a drug that won't be approved by the FDA. Are fat people so disposable, their quality of life considered so unbearable, that a premature death as a result of taking a dangerous drug is a risk worth taking to stimulate this business?

The fact is, fatness is a result of a multitude of factors, some of which may be biological, environmental, and behavioral, the order and composition of which differ for pretty much everyone. There is no magic bullet to "cure" fatness because we simply don't understand it well enough.

In February of 2011, the FDA formally rejected Contrave's bid for approval, citing the potential risks to heart health, and as predicted, this move has likely killed obesity research for the forseeable future. If drug companies with millions of dollars in research funding and the smartest brains in all the land, inspired by the prospect of untold profits if they can find a diet drug that actually works—if these powerhouses cannot solve the "problem" of obesity, maybe there is no solution, or maybe obesity is not really a problem at all.

The Jenny Craig weight-loss center I knew was located in one of the blank-faced strip malls that make up a majority of the commercial architecture where I grew up. South Florida is a place where impermanence is part of the culture—the result of the collective influence of hurricanes, tourism, and retirees. This atmosphere of change persists today in storefront plastic surgery shops, where you can buy a new shape or a more expressionless face on your lunch hour.

The furnishings inside the Jenny Craig store were white, all straight lines and ninety-degree angles, a model of sterile late-1980s design. At my request, my father had brought me here, supplying both transportation and payment. Though I did learn some of my food issues from my family, I never remember my father being anything other than quietly supportive of my dieting efforts, and I never remember him making me feel badly about the money spent—or wasted—when I inevitably failed to lose weight. The woman at the reception desk was dark haired, with a mask-like smile. She handed me a few forms on a plastic clipboard, and a pen. I sat in one of the armless chairs in the waiting area and wrote out the pertinent details of my short life. I was thirteen.

There was a hopefulness to this process; I'd felt it before. It was the promise of a new start, the proverbial clean slate, like procuring new notebooks and pens at the beginning of the school year and feeling the vastness of possibility. This year I would do better, I would rise above my middle school social problems and get better grades. I would be smarter and better and happier and everything would change. This was the year. And like every diet before, this was *the* diet—the one that would save me. A well-trained consumer, I knew by now that I could be changed by the things I purchased, even with my father's money. I could not be trusted to consume food, but I could consume diets. I could acquire something to make me different, better. Jenny Craig would be the answer, because all of its food came in boxes purchased at the center. It offered an endless cycle of shopping for redemption.

I followed the woman who would be my counselor back into the maze of narrow corridors and tiny rooms. She wore a white coat with all the vague confidence of a person who has no medical training whatsoever— and indeed she was not a medical professional, though she could play one here—and ushered me into a small room with a desk and a cabinet. Everything was white, reminiscent of a doctor's office.

My counselor explained the process. First, I would

diet to lose weight. Then, I would be taught to eat appropriately on my own, without the aid of all my food boxes from Jenny Craig. Finally, I would enter the "maintenance phase," which would be the point after the loss where I would rejoin the eating world. Delicately, with care and restraint. Fact is, I could not envision a point beyond the weight loss, even then, but she sounded so hopeful and positive, I trusted that she knew what would happen. Frankly I was more interested in the diet than the future; I was more interested in penance than salvation.

The counselor led me out of the room and had me stand at the far end of the hallway. She took my picture using a Polaroid instant camera with a supernova-level flash that blasted all the image's detail into a high-contrast haze. And I smiled, because I was a kid and I knew that when someone points a camera at you, your task is to smile.

Though I have not seen it since 1990, I remember the image with a precision that is ummatched by most of my other memories from the same time period. I remember watching my shape develop and appear from a pale square of shining film edged in white. In it, I am standing slightly off center, my back to the institutional gray wall behind me, like a suspect in a line-up. My face bears a half-formed smile, as though the shutter went too soon; my expression is nevertheless positive, hopeful, eager. The shirt I wear is by a clothing company called Ultra Pink: long sleeved, screen printed with a French-themed collage of random words and the Eiffel Tower, in purple, green, and black, dusted with sequins at points in the design deserving of extra attention. It is cut long and voluminous around the midsection, which is a reassurance to me, even though I have yet to reach the point at which I am regularly sized out of non-plus shops. I have paired this shirt with purple knit stirrup pants from Lerner's, and cheap Payless ballet flats decorated with huge puffy bows that I bought with my allowance.

The Polaroid was to be my "before" picture. The counselor took it with an impressive measure of enthusiasm, with an absolute wide-eyed assurance that someday soon I would look at this picture and shake my head and say, "I cannot believe I ever looked like that!" This Polaroid was paperclipped to my file at Jenny Craig, and every time I went in for my weekly weigh-in and counseling session, I would see it there, clipped to the folder, like a piece of my soul.

I was wearing roughly a size sixteen at this time, and when placed on the scale, I weighed 168 pounds, which was recorded by the counselor as the beginning point on my weight-loss line chart. The shape of the handwritten number at the first column persists in my memory like a scar, inclining right, tidy and legible; every year in elementary school I got A's in everything except penmanship, which often earned me a C. My handwriting was thoughtless, slovenly, unpredictable, like my body. That prim 168 represented the changes in myself I was seeking to make, to become neat, identifiable, understood, normal. We were seated on opposite sides of the cheap white desk in the counseling room, and my counselor produced a tape measure and wrapped it around my wrist: seven inches. She was impressed by the number. *Does this mean I really do have big bones?* She instructed me that the target weight for my height and my wrist measurement was a generous 130 pounds.

Staring at me from under the paper clip in my file was my own picture, taken minutes ago. I looked at that girl and had a brief moment in which I felt desperately sorry for her. She looked nice enough. Why did she have to be so fat? I was flooded with regret, not for the choice of diet but for the picture, for allowing this place to capture and keep me in that photograph. The Jenny Craig center had an entire wall of Polaroids, befores matched with afters, demonstrating clients' success. The befores were so sad to me, like discarded skins. But I did not hate myself. I could not. Whether as a result of my nature or the circumstances of my life thus far, I appreciated myself, my strength and resourcefulness and intelligence. I just didn't want to be picked on in school anymore.

We finished my consultation, and they sent me off with good wishes and an astonishing number of blue-and-white boxes of food that would comprise my diet for the foreseeable future. The boxes were an embarrassment of riches, representing a relief that I would no longer have to think about the foods I ate. Everything was already decided, prepared, meted out, and I would merely follow instructions. These boxes would change me, would repair my brokenness. These things we had purchased would redefine my life and my body, reshape me into something real, something true. They would reveal the authentic body within the fat body that was crushing me.

I asked my father what he remembered of this experience. "I actually signed up with you," he told me, "and lost a bunch of weight right away, and I remember feeling guilty because you didn't." Pause. "Also, I remember it was very expensive."

For the first few weeks the line on my chart edged its way downhill and my imminent slenderness seemed as inevitable as gravity. All I needed to do was obey the rules, eat from the boxes, and keep my whims and desires bounded within Jenny's small blue-and-white world. I was disciplined, and my body began to slide away, pound by pound, until even the clerk at the grocery store—where I selected supplemental items like romaine lettuce, red wine vinegar, and pickles—was remarking on my changing size.

After a couple months of adherence, I had lost around fifteen pounds. Then the chart's steady downward slope leveled out. After the first week that I didn't lose weight, my counselor was sympathetic. The second week, she attempted to explain that sometimes people losing weight will hit something called a plateau, in which their loss is stalled for a period of time. It was an apt description of the line on my chart, which had flattened out well above the alleged paradise I was hoping to reach. Her solution was to diet through the plateau, promising me that it would end and the loss would then continue.

It didn't occur to me to question the science behind this idea, behind any of it. I was thirteen.

The only thing that had kept me loyal to Jenny's wise counsel was my continuing weight loss. So as the weight loss stuttered to a halt, my devotion began to wane. Why eat from boxes if there is no reward and the food is terrible? And the food was *terrible*. I don't know if things have changed in the interim but at the time, some of the boxed meals were practically inedible, like a vague approximation of food designed by an alien who has observed people eating but has never actually had the experience. Years later, when I taste something that reminds me of the food I ate while faithful to Jenny, the reaction is traumatic. I remember the rubbery pancakes, sickeningly sweet with artificial sugars, the pizza with the texture of plastic melted over cardboard, the brittle dehydrated pasta salad. The memory makes me nauseous and sad.

As my weight loss faltered, I began to zero in on the few Jenny Craig food items that tasted at all pleasurable to me, the most memorable of which were something called peanut butter bars, which consisted of a crumbly and dry peanut-like bar encased in a brown substance meant to evoke memories of chocolate, if not chocolate itself. It tasted better than the alternatives, almost like a treat, and I was by this time operating under a near-constant obsession with my never-fully-satisfied hunger. I would sneak extra peanut butter bars. I was meant to have one a day, for a snack, but then I started eating two, and soon it was more still. I began to crave them, likely because they were the option highest in fat and sugar.

The standard human biological response to starvation (by diet or otherwise) is a craving for sweets, as sugars are most readily processed into energy when our reserves are running low. Dieters know these cravings well. Indeed, as a child I never liked sweets or candy, and would routinely refuse birthday cake at parties in favor of the vegetable tray. I only started to seek out sugar once I began dieting.

My counselor began to get suspicious when I was telling her I needed another box of these precious peanut butter bars every week. Part of her job, arguably the most important part, was to keep track of what foods I had bought and what I reordered. She never really counseled me, in the sense that the commercials seem to describe, by patting my hand, listening to my woes, or being my confidante for half an hour once a week. She was primarily a gatekeeper. "If you're following the plan, you should have plenty of these at home," she scolded when I insisted I needed more bars, peering at me with undisguised annoyance.

I knew what she thought, and I knew what it meant because I had thought it too. *So it's your fault you can't get off the plateau.* My internal monologue took the shape of unspoken accusations from my Jenny Craig counselor. *Here I am working for you, believing in you, and you are letting us down. You are letting everyone down, too weak to resist the slightest temptation, to follow the simplest plan. You eat from the boxes, you lose the weight, that's how it goes. If you don't, the failure is yours.*

I stayed on the plateau for a couple weeks more before I told my father I didn't want to go anymore, and that was that. He never pressured me to keep to it, and the grocery clerk stopped making approving comments about my body, which slowly recollected what I had lost and returned to its prior shape.

And Jenny Craig still had my photograph.

This knowledge was nearly unbearable. I felt as though I had surrendered a piece of myself to Jenny's promises of success, and when I failed, apparently because of my own weakness, I felt an urge to erase any evidence that it had ever happened. I wanted to retrieve the optimism I'd felt when I first signed up, the day they backed me up against the wall as if facing a firing squad, the whole of Jenny's high-priced weaponry aimed at my hated fat, and took my picture. This was not my first diet failure and it would not be my last, but I came away from each more bitter, beaten down, and hopeless. I couldn't spare any more hope. I couldn't waste what little I had left. I wanted that photograph back.

I told myself stories about getting it. Depending on the circumstances, and how brazen I was feeling, sometimes I would break into the strip mall Jenny Craig in the dead of night, imagining myself rifling though drawers with one hand, holding a flashlight with the other. Sometimes I would march in during business hours, full of purpose and rage, and demand they retrieve the photo from my file. While the employees scurried around in a dither, terrified by my righteous anger, I would dryly warn the new recruits in the waiting room that they'd be better off eating their money than spending it there.

The likely reality was that the center kept my information on file for a certain period of time, expecting me to come back. Even the failures often return; it's not for nothing that Jenny Craig and Weight Watchers both offer lifetime membership options, under which clients are allowed to come back as often as they like for a long as they are alive. Simple logic would dictate that if the program truly worked, such lifetime commitments would not be necessary, but you see, it's not Jenny who fails. It's you.

So I imagine I lived on, a Polaroid ghost, in the files of my local Jenny storefront for some time. Eventually I would have been culled as a lost cause, my file destroyed, my picture thrown away. In a landfill somewhere in Florida there lies a chart with a bold "168" written on it, followed by a line in short decline, followed by a long straight plateau, and a picture of a slightly chubby thirteen-year-old with an aching smile, a moment of desperate longing captured, and then buried forever.

Back in the early aughts, I started giving campus talks and lectures on fat politics. I used a seminar format that involved lots of questions and participation from the audience, and conversations would occasionally get sidetracked.The usual culprit? A not-fat girl either suffering from or in recovery for an eating disorder (ED).

So when I'd get halfway through my talk about fatness (and the lack thereof) in popular media, and inevitably someone in the room would raise her hand and start disclosing her ED, it posed a unique problem. How do I redirect this conversation without dismissing this woman's experience and her desire to share it? That is important! We should talk about eating disorders and body image issues freely and without shame. I wanted to support people with eating disorders without allowing that subject to dominate my discussion, which was supposed to be about fat.

Of course, the fat body and the eating-disordered body are related issues. The writer Susan Bordo has said, "The obese and the anoretic are therefore disturbing partly because they embody resistance to cultural norms." In the anoretic body, this embodiment is an illustration of what happens when our rules about restriction and denial are taken to dramatic lengths. In the obese body, we see a reflection of what can happen when those rules are disregarded altogether.

In lived experience though, being fat is very different from being not-fat but having an ED (also different is being fat and having an ED at the same time, which happens in spite of our lack of context for it). There are many ways in which these issues differ, and they are not necessarily two sides of the same coin, as is often presumed. The experience of *feeling* fat and hating your body, may share aspects in common with actually *being* fat. But being fat brings with it some other baggage that a non-fat person cannot reconcile. It's one thing to look in the mirror and see yourself as a huge and hideous monster. It's another thing to fear going out to eat because you're not sure if you'll fit in the booth with your friends. Both are tragic. But they are different.

Further, it is no more acceptable to make assumptions about the eating and exercise habits of a person with a fat body than it is of a thin one, though this happens to members of both groups. But body types are not infallible indicators of daily practices. There is a quote often attributed to Marilyn Wann, one of the best-known fat activists, that goes something like this: "the only thing you can tell for sure by looking at a fat person is your own degree of bias against fat people."

Fat people are culturally depicted as not knowing how to eat correctly, that is, for sustenance and nothing more. They're emotional eaters, you know, because it is abnormal, even pathological to eat food simply because it tastes good or is comforting. But isn't all eating emotional for everyone on some level? The disorders of binge eating and compulsive overeating—chronically misapplied to all fat folks—are an addiction model used to explain behavior and describe their sufferers as being literally addicted to food. However, fat people are subject to all variations of eating habits and disorders, including anorexia. The actual number of fat people with eating disorders is unknown, as too often these practices are registered simply as diets. Technically, fat people can't be diagnosed with anorexia no matter their degree of self-starvation because one of the diagnostic criterion is a failure to maintain at least 85 percent of expected body weight for height and age. This does not stop fat anoretics who meet every other criterion from exhibiting this eating disorder.

Pro-anorexia (often shortened to pro-ana) is an ideology that argues in favor of eating disorders as a legitimate lifestyle choice. Though the "pro-ana" shorthand specifies anorexia, it is generally applied to any eating-disordered behavior. Lazy thinkers sometimes attempt to link fat acceptance communities with pro-ana ones as equally irresponsible and dangerous movements. It might seem like a neat and tidy thing to build a spectrum with extreme fatness and extreme thinness on either end, in a perfectly balanced analogy. The problem is that eating disorders are behavior, not body type, and while fat politics advocate for the acceptability of a certain body type, they do not systematically advocate for overeating, which would be necessary for this analogy to work. What pro-ana groups do share with fat acceptance communities is the finding of beauty in body shapes considered ugly by conventional standards, as well as a desire for full bodily autonomy, unrestrained by well-meaning arbiters. But there the similarities end.

Pro-ana resources often describe anorexic behaviors as the natural extension of a weight-loss diet, and they're not far off the mark. Self-induced starvation may be a symptom of an ED, but it is not only that; nor is it simply a funhouse-mirror distortion of "healthy" habits. It is an accurate reflection of our culture around eating and food. We feel its pressure everywhere we go. It touches every one of us, this compulsion toward control, this unwillingness to trust our hunger, to have faith in our bodies' inclination toward survival, and to live in concert with our needs. Our bodies are anarchists, we think! Our bodies are out to destroy us by accumulating fat we don't want, by putting it in places we'd rather it not go, by constantly demanding food, care, attention, nourishment, energy that we can't spare. Our bodies are described as wild horses to be broken, to be saddled and bridled and worn down. Our nature is chaotic and not to be trusted. Managing this requires constant vigilance and never "letting go"—never ever can you "let yourself go." Chaos would ensue. While our bodies are demanding food, our culture is educating us on the terrible dangers of allowing our needs and desires take their own course and on the moral implications of failing to keep them in check.

The reality is that fat people are often supported in hating their bodies, in starving themselves, in engaging in unsafe exercise, and in seeking out weight loss by any means necessary. A thin person who does these things is considered mentally ill. A fat person who does these things is redeemed by them. This is why our culture has no concept of a fat person who also has an eating disorder. If you're fat, it's not an eating disorder—it's a *lifestyle change.*

Pro-anorexia thinking makes perfect sense in the context in which we all live and eat. Weight-loss-based reality television series are enormously popular, and publicly reward those who cast all caution to the wind in a single-minded effort to be thin. While individual ED sufferers have individual circumstances, as a cultural phenomenon eating disorders are the product of overwhelming pressure to meticulously defend our bodies against our own needs. This pressure breaks us. It takes the normal impulses for eating and hunger and shatters them into a thousand unrecognizable pieces.

A culture that supports weight loss by any means necessary is a culture that supports eating disorders. It is a culture that supports the sickening and weakening of us all, in the name of improving our health, the very thing that we sacrifice. It instructs us either to succeed or be destroyed by the effort. Our reaction, socially, to eating disorders tends to be one of fear and disgust. But this is what diet culture has created. By making eating disorders shameful, we isolate the very people who are in greatest need of support.

To some extent, eating disorders are a compulsive urge to control the uncontrollable—one might as well try to lasso the ocean. At a certain point, we don't have intellectual control over our bodies any longer, no matter how hard we try, no matter how fierce our conviction. The only way to win the fight with our bodies is to die, as everyone must, inevitably do, no matter their size or their state of health. So much of the rhetoric found in fat hatred and diet culture focuses on the idea that fat people die, as though thin people don't. But we can't go on starving ourselves, and starving each other, and expect anyone to survive.

I n January of 2001, I was beginning the final semester of my first master's degree. One wintry eve late in the month, I started to feel unwell. Six hours later I was in such indescribable, excruciating pain that I thought I was dying. Or else about to end a brief sojourn as host to a baby alien growing inside the right upper quadrant of my torso.

Having spent several hours vomiting bile and doubled over in an unusually precise sensation of abdominal pain, I finally realized something was very wrong. Around six that morning, I woke my partner and told him to take me to the hospital.

I was seen right away. The emergency room doctor took one withering look at me, curtly pronounced the culprit as "gastroenteritis," and left. I knew he was wrong but lacked the ability to argue. I spent a few hours being rehydrated by IV, the doctor visibly annoyed by my insistence on vomiting up even water. *It's just gastroenteritis, you big baby*, I imagined him thinking, disgusted.

I went to my primary care doctor the following week to discover what had really happened. She sent me for an ultrasound, and there I saw my blurry gall-bladder, filled with stones rattling around like bits of gravel as I shifted position per the instructions of the ultrasound technician. It gives me a shiver even to remember it—there is an unnamable horror that goes along with seeing things happening inside your own body, things going awry that you cannot control. So it was gallstones. The gallbladder had to come out.

I was confused by my apparent need to exorcise my gallbladder. I was young, and gallbladder problems requiring surgery are uncommon in those under sixty. I was a strict vegetarian and had been for several years, and vegetarians virtually never get gallstones (fiber is an enemy of gallstones, and the typical vegetarian diet is fiber heavy; diets high in animal fat and cholesterol are gallstone-friendly, and vegetarians consume little or no animal-based foods). The only clue as to the cause of my condition came from a nurse who asked, "Have you done a lot of dieting?" The answer was yes.

Due to the vulgarities of health insurance, I could not have this procedure done in Boston, where I was attending that all-important final semester of my master's program, without which I would not get my degree. I had to have the surgery done in Florida, where my father still lived, off whose health insurance I was sponging as a full-time graduate student. I needed to graduate on time, so I would have to wait to have my gallbladder exorcised until the semester was over. I would have to live with this problem for four months, which required me to learn what it was that angered my rogue gallbladder and avoid those things at all costs.

Turns out, there are many foods that can upset dodgy gallbladders, and they are often different for every body. Dietary fat is often a common culprit, as the gallbladder is the body's bile warehouse, and bile is instrumental for the digestion of fats. Thus, when we eat fatty foods, the gallbladder gets worked up, and if you have the misfortune of playing host to a sadistic jerk of a gallbladder, pain of varying degrees can result.

Hence, the thing that most enraged my gallbladder was, predictably, fat. As a vegetarian the only fats I ate were plant based, but apparently that was also the culprit. It was, in fact, a meal of zucchini roasted with a bit of olive oil that triggered the first attack. While my gallbladder could peacefully abide the fat on my body, it violently revolted against any fat I swallowed, inhaled, absorbed, or otherwise inserted into my digestive tract. This much was clear.

I don't exaggerate when I describe how painful this first attack was. It was a memorable pain. The kind of pain where one longs for unconsciousness. Seared-into-your-mind-for-all-time pain. Later, I would observe that I'd always assumed there was a limit to the degree of pain a person can feel before they pass out. This limit may well exist, but it is much less conservative than I had thought. The memory of that pain is no small thing.

Because I so desperately feared a repeat performance of what brought me to the emergency room, I decided that for the next four months I would go on the most fat-restrictive diet I could muster. I would eat no fat at all. I subsisted for that period on apples, potatoes, brown rice, various beans and legumes, and tomato-and-lettuce sandwiches on fat-free bread with fat-free mayonnaise. I fell back into the routine of food restriction easily, robotically, as though the programming was still there, the discipline had never left. It was merely waiting to be reactivated.

I was always a very good dieter, at least until my efforts stopped producing a measureable effect. In this case, however, the desired outcome was not weight loss, but rather a lack of debilitating pain. With that for motivation, I was monk-like in my restriction: dedicated, single-minded, chop wood, carry water, eat before you pass out. I ate as little as possible and what I did eat was swallowed with all the pleasure of shoveling coal into a furnace. I ate purely for the purpose of surviving long enough to have my surgery and regain the ability to eat normally again.

I finished my degree four months later. I went to Florida the following day.

I arrived at the hospital in the morning and underwent the necessary preparations. There was an unexpected delay, during which I lay in the pre-surgery ward for two hours, terrified, wearing only a hospital gown, my resolve melting, my partner trying to keep me engaged, a nurse having drugged me with something—valium?—that she said would make me feel as though I'd had a glass of wine. It did make me drowsy, but my anxiety skyrocketed, adrenaline surging, realizing if I had to fight my way out of the hospital (I might!) then it would be all the more difficult to do with this slow muck in my veins. (When she came around with the syringe a second time, I declined.) Eventually I had to go to the bathroom, and there I was, a freeze-frame from a million sitcoms, wobbling unsteadily down a corridor, carrying my IV bag in one hand and with my bare-ass behind swinging in the sterile air, defying the weak protestations of the open-backed hospital robe.

My partner helped me, but stopped at the bathroom door to give me some privacy. I did my business and when I rose to flush I realized I'd been holding the IV bag too low, causing my blood to back up into the long and narrow connecting tube running from the back of my hand to the bag of fluid, turning it from clear and antiseptic to red-black and ominous. I nearly lost my bearings then, seeing my blood snaking in wisps into that IV bag. I opened the door and told my partner, "I messed it up," or something like that and then wordlessly showed him the tube with my blood in it, where it wasn't supposed to go. My partner gallantly took the IV bag from me and hefted it high, and my blood came back in. He walked me back to the hospital bed where I would continue to wait.

There was a point, minutes before they brought me in for the surgery, at which I could not manage my fear and rage anymore, and I cried. I said, "Why can't they just get on with it?"

The anesthesiologist, whom I'd met a few days before, told me that once I was put under, there'd be no time, no awareness. I'd had tubes in my ears twice as a kid, and I remembered the vivid dreams I had during those minor procedures. But no, with this sort of anesthesia there'd be none of that. He said, "It will feel as though you've just closed your eyes, and then opened them again."

They wheeled me down the hall to the operating room. Things seemed to go very fast, and I felt very slow. The mask came down; it wasn't secure on my face and I tried to tell him, "It's not . . . "

I closed my eyes.

I opened my eyes.

Well, except I didn't. I tried to open them but couldn't; they were taped shut. My eyes rolled fruitlessly against my eyelids, and I could hear the room, and had an odd sensory awareness of the space, but I could not move anything else. I spiked into a terrible panic and immediately heard multiple voices telling me to calm down. It's just the anesthesia. I couldn't listen; clearly they didn't understand that I couldn't fucking move and if anything was worth panicking over, that was. But then, all at once, I could feel my muscles again.

It was only after they'd wheeled me out of the operating room that I realized the surgery must be over.

In recovery, they brought me ice and a giant white

elastic band, at least ten inches wide, to wrap around and compress my midsection. It was too small, far too small, but the nurse heaved and pulled—me apologizing groggily as she did so (for my girth? my inability to assist?)—and she managed to secure it. Velcro. Another nurse came by and noted that the compression band seemed to be too small. I murmured, "I doubt I am the fattest person ever to have my gallbladder removed." She said they'd find me a larger one, but she never came back.

My throat hurt. Someone mentioned that it was because of the tube. *Why did they put a tube in my throat*, I wondered. I was beginning to grasp that my body had gone on some strange adventure without me. My brain choked off, my voice eclipsed. A heap of meat on an operating table, one in an assembly line of common surgeries.

I'd begun to look at fat politics four years prior to this surgery. It's been a long process, and if it's not a long process for you then you may be doing it wrong, or else you just may not realize when it began. I had stopped trying to lose weight. I had come to love myself, uneasily, and to live in a truce with my body, if not in contentment or pleasure. I was tolerant of my body; we shared a loveless marriage that was nevertheless comfortable and secure.

But lying in the recovery ward, I realized these things had happened to my body and I hadn't been there. It was as though the whole of my history of body-hatred and self-punishment rose up on me like a towering black monolith, all at once, and I came to realize the immensity of the damage I'd done, the disdain I'd held for myself, my body, my health, during my years of self-induced deprivation. The only real risk factor I had for the gallstones was a long history of weight cycling and yo-yo dieting. I thought, *What did I do all that for? Why did I work so hard to beat up the awesome vessel that brings me to the world?*

My surgery was straightforward and complication-free. I had expected, hilariously in retrospect, that this was an outpatient procedure, that I'd have the surgery and a few hours later I would go home. I don't know why I believed this. I don't know why no one corrected me beforehand. I was never told anything, in advance or after, about what to expect and I never asked.

Overnight I would face gruesome pain as the anesthesia wore off, but my pain tolerance is legendary and I knew that all I had to do was hang on until the morning. My partner stayed with me, sleeping uncomfortably in a chair beside my bed, heroically ignoring his own fear of hospitals born of childhood operations. I could be strong for him. I watched television. When it got so late that nothing was on, I read Maya Angelou's *I Know Why the Caged Bird Sings* for the first time, straight through, and when I finally nodded into light sleep I dreamed of my gallbladder literally sprouting wings and taking flight from the cage of my body.

Around 10:30 that morning, a little more than twenty-four hours after I'd arrived, I was sent home to my father's house to convalesce for a full week, which I did with all the patience and care that you might expect—that is, none at all. But I healed and returned to my home in Boston and, most importantly, returned to eating normally.

I had a follow-up appointment with my local primary care doctor a couple of weeks following the surgery, by which point I'd been easing myself back into eating my usual array of foods—cheese had never tasted so good. I attended the appointment like the dutiful patient I am, but it was primarily because I was curious about one thing: I wanted to see how much weight I had lost on the gallbladder diet. I presumed that four months of extreme restriction had to count for something and I was curious to see what effects the most radical diet of my life would have. I was aware of the little self-destructive impulses this sort of thinking fired off in my brain but I ignored them. I had to have lost weight, surely! I mentioned this to my doctor as I approached the scale. She smiled and nodded and I stepped up.

Three pounds.

I'd lost three pounds.

Four months of the most restrictive diet, a diet conceived in terrifying pain and reinforced by the fear of that pain being inflicted again. A diet I did not even for a moment contemplate cheating on, or deviating from. Three pounds. It wasn't that the diet should have "worked." It was that I still believed it would work for me. I still thought I could diet myself skinny, if I just had the discipline to do it. But those three pounds were a revelation—it was in that instant that everything crystallized. I got it. I got fat politics, like some folks get religion. All at once. *I see it now. I am fat.*

And as this realization was swirling around in my head, I could hear my doctor speaking, as though she was far away, her voice saying brightly, "Well, I think that's a great start on the road you have ahead of you." The road to slenderness, to a "normal" body. But I was off to a different start.

I still feel sad for my gallbladder, a lost child forever wandering the bodily organ version of Neverland, maybe hand-in-hand (duct-in-duct?) with the other innocent gallbladders parted from their abdominal homes too soon. I never meant to hurt myself so badly. At the time I thought of my compulsive crash diets as open-handed slaps to my hated fatness, not the kind of deep trauma that could ever result in long-term damage. I made mistakes. I suffered the consequences.

More than that, however, I emerged from this experience more ferociously in favor of body acceptance and self-love than ever before. I felt, vividly, the importance of owning one's body and living in it fully, and realized that all the abuse we heap upon ourselves does take a toll, be it emotional or physical. I came to understand for the first time ever the importance of being healthy, and I don't mean the universalizing and troubling concept of "diet conscious" our culture currently prefers, but the kind of healthy that encourages and cultivates a knowledge and awareness of your unique body and what it can be reasonably asked to do, and to never feel shame if your body does not operate by the same rules as someone else's body. I'm talking about a healthy that is rooted in self-determination and individual autonomy, and is thus applicable to a spectrum of bodies, including professional athletes, cancer survivors, gym rats, the doctor-phobic, the poor, joggers, and folks with a limited supply of spoons, a healthy that excludes no one and that is specific and relative to the individual.

Why did I starve myself? Why did I diet? Why did I relish deprivation as the source of my salvation? Because I thought it would make me happy. It did not. It took a childhood and adolescence of failed diets and a surgery that I might have avoided to make me see that this was not the road to contentment. It was a vicious cycle of the same shit, the same failures, the same guilt over and over again, never going anywhere but around and around.

Finally, I was able to say: no more.

I t wasn't until I was in my twenties that I knew what fat community was like. In 2003, I saw the formation of a new group, hosted on the online diary site LiveJournal, where I was an active participant. The community was created by Amanda Piasecki, an artist, social justice activist, community-organizing genius, and fat-style rock star. Amanda called the community Fatshionista. She created Fatshionista as a dedicated forum for conversations about fashion, culture, and subculture, knowing that there were people in our friends' extended communities who would positively contribute. She was interested in "coming out" about the day-to-day realities of living in a fat body with hopes of dispelling shame, sharing resources, and creating a better quality of life for the fat people in her community.

I had experienced some degree of fat-positive community in small doses before Fatshionista, but this was an entirely new experience for me. The early membership was radical through and through, and every one of the early posts was replete with a sense of relief and joy at having a space to discuss the challenges of fat fashion without making the obligatory sacrifices to the conventional wisdom around fat bodies—that they are temporary, shameful, and ought to be invisible. The first rule was "no fat hatred allowed." The space was intimate and self-selective.

I was finishing my second master's degree and ultimately leaving academia, where I'd been having similar conversations always from the perspective of the token fatty, the one person speaking up for fat bodies in broader conversations about representation. These conversations were challenging and critical; if we complained about a lack of plus-size models in clothing catalogs, we also talked about the profit-driven nature of such enterprises. If we shared our struggles with effectively thrifting plus-size clothing, we also discussed the class implications and the reality that while thrifting is a fun diversion for some, it is an absolute necessity for others. An early requirement was that for every bit of fluff in a post, there had to be an entry point for critical discussion.

Within the first year, however, things began to change. A massive, heterogeneous membership joined the forum—over eight thousand and counting, as of this writing—and discussions became more about self-acceptance and personal transformation and less about politics and community.

When I came on board as a Fatshionista moderator around six months after its creation, I never would have believed I would remain there for six years, but I was thrilled that a community I so loved wanted to include me in such a way. This job—unpaid as it was—was a responsibility that could be both thankless and rewarding. With the community's growth, the conversations that were once respectful and productive chats between people who were politically aligned became intense fights with newer members who sought the community out not as a place for political discussion but as a guide to find decent clothes to wear. Of course, the beauty of such happy accidents is that a great many members who came to the community just looking for pants that fit would later become some of its most compelling supporters.

Community is transformative. It is all the more so when the community is built around something that we are not supposed to be—something that is culturally abhorrent. We draw strength from sharing experiences that otherwise leave us isolated, and from sharing an understanding of things that are unrepresented in the predominant culture. In fat community, these things can be a love of horizontal stripes or a predilection for fat sexual partners, a passion for belly dancing or a commitment to fat-friendly yoga. The reason we respond with such euphoria at finding a community that understands us is that it gives us permission to be who we want to be. It validates our longings and hidden desires. A supportive community provides camaraderie and strength against the cultural forces that tell us no, no, no.

As a terrified fourteen-year-old digging through the boxes of school uniforms, I had no community, no one who would understand, and as a result I felt utterly alone. In a typically egocentric teenager way, I was convinced that I was the only person this had ever happened to, that I was the fattest person ever to attend private school, that it was all my fault and that I therefore deserved my isolation and shame. I could not speak of it to anyone because more than anything I feared their pity. I didn't want to be pathetic. I wanted someone to say, "Oh yes, I know how that is, I went through it too." Or better, "Oh yes, and what bullshit it is that no one asked you your size first or helped you to find something to fit." This longing to be understood is a part of the human condition, for all of us, but when your experience is less common, the likelihood of finding like-minded folks is less as well.

Fortunately today we have the internet, and communities like Fatshionista, and all the ones that will come after it, that are filled with the relief and gratitude of new members who thought they were alone. I've heard it argued that fat-positive communities, both structured ones like Fatshionista and more loosely defined groups like the fat blogosphere, are dangerous because they glorify obesity, but this is a misunderstanding of both the concept of glorification and of what fat-acceptance communities seek to do. Glorifying obesity implies that we aspire to some kind of superiority—as if wanting a decent selection of well-fitting clothing, fair treatment in medical settings, and to be given the same respect and dignity of non-fat people is simply taking things too far. Glorifying suggests that fat people have no right to basic access that non-fat people take for granted, and that giving them that access would be unfairly elevating their status over the people who get these privileges as a matter of course.

Fat people have always existed, and will never be eradicated from the persistent diversity of human forms. In community, we can be strong, and when we are weak we can lean on each other for support. The prevailing cultural ideology tells us that fat bodies are unnatural and abhorrent, the sign of a weak will or gluttonous nature. Fat-positive spaces and communities take this idea on, a juggernaut of fat realities barreling against the tide, saying, we exist, we have each other, and you cannot wipe us away.

When I was eight years old, around the same time that I was first becoming aware of my size and the fact that my body was bigger and had a belly when my friends' bodies did not, I loved unicorns. No, that is putting it too delicately. I was obsessed with unicorns, in the all-encompassing way that only a small girl in the mid-1980s could be. My room was decorated with unicorn posters. All my school folders were unicorn-emblazoned. I spent countless hours reading about unicorns in books from the library. I could close my eyes and visualize an army of unicorns as perfectly as if they were standing in neat rows before me. I was past the age when I still believed in Santa Claus, but I knew unicorns were real. I *knew.* I knew someday I'd find one, a massive, muscular white horse with a flowing mane and a single glimmering, spiraling horn. My unicorn would be able to talk and would become my best friend. My imaginary unicorn friend would occasionally have wings, because I very much liked the idea of a unicorn who could fly.

How I would find my own special unicorn was beyond me. I was aware that, although unicorns absolutely positively did exist, they were very, very rare. I expected I would find mine purely by virtue of my unwavering conviction. So long as I believed that magical meeting would happen, it would. So long as I trusted in the legend and kept the faith, I would not miss my chance to make it come true.

In 1985, the circus came to town. Every time the circus came to town, my father would take me to see it. But while the circus itself was not an unusual event, this year there was something new, something remarkable, something I would never forget. This year, the circus would be exhibiting the world's only living unicorn.

Oh, you can try to imagine my excitement. My father, who was intimately aware of my unicorn fasci-

nation, shared in my enthusiasm, and built the anticipation daily leading up to the big event.

The circus day came. I sat in my place on the
bleachers under the tent and waited with my father
beside me. It was noisy and hot, and smelled of mil-
dew and elephant dung, but I barely noticed. I was all
on pins and needles, waiting for them to reveal the
unicorn, waiting for the moment when all my faith
would be justified. I remember almost nothing of that
particular circus save my anxious anticipatory fidgeting. And then finally the moment came. A float came
out and circled the arena slowly, a float bedecked with
all manner of dazzling decorations building to a peak,
like a tiny rolling mountain, and at the top were two
unicorn tenders and . . . the unicorn.

Except it was not a unicorn.

The brilliant white stallion of my daydreams was
missing, as was the glimmering spiral horn. Instead, I
saw a large, long-haired white goat, with a single thick
and cylindrical horn, painted gold, perched awkwardly
on its head.

For a moment, I tried to believe. I felt a flicker of
panic as I struggled to comprehend what was taking
place. I tried very hard to squint and make it real. But I
just couldn't do it in the face of this damning evidence.
It was not a unicorn. I didn't need an expert opinion. I

didn't need a genetic profile or a peer-reviewed study of the origins of the animal on top of that float. I could see it with my own eyes, right there, in front of me, in three dimensions. Fake. The unicorn was a lie.

My heart was broken. My father leaned down and jostled me, "Look, sweetheart, it's your unicorn!" Not wanting to disappoint him, I smiled and said, "Yes, yes, it's beautiful, Dad."

But I knew. I knew then that unicorns weren't real, as inexorably as I had believed that they were only moments before. If unicorns were real, the circus would have no reason to create a fake one—and an appallingly bad fake one at that. Unicorns were a myth, and always had been, whether I believed in them or not. I cried, quietly.

I mourned for weeks afterward, keening silently over the loss of my belief, over the realization that simply wishing for something doesn't make it so, no matter how hard I wish.

The moral of this story—the moral I'd share with anyone still fighting to become a fantasy self, still struggling to believe that they are exclusively and personally responsible for their failures to force their bodies into a certain shape, to fit an arbitrary beauty ideal, to satisfy the fairytale ending in which the heroine loses the weight and lives happily ever after—the moral is this: *Unicorns aren't real.*

It hurts, I know. It hurts to let it go. It hurts because of all you've invested in that belief. All the effort, the conviction, the sacrifice. I know. I know how realizing that my circus unicorn was a fake ripped through my tiny eight-year-old soul. I know how coming to terms with the fact that I will never, ever look like a model— even a plus-size model—was a brutal and excruciating reckoning and frequently sent me into spirals of self-loathing and despair, even for a long time after I thought I was over it. *I know.* But unicorns aren't real. And trying to believe that they are, even in the face of convincing evidence to the contrary, is both futile and a disservice to yourself.

The world doesn't need unicorns for me to see beauty and magic in it. And as I get to demonstrate to myself daily, I don't need to meet a certain standard of slenderness in order to be a happy, healthy, satisfied individual with a fabulous life. Though it may not have been the one I'd set my sights on originally, that's the truth I've earned. And I can live with that.

ACKNOWLEDGMENTS

Thank you to Dennis Scimeca, Marianne Kirby, and Hanne Blank, for being my unfailing support system throughout the process of writing this book. You are constant sources of inspiration and wise counsel, and I couldn't have done it without you. Thank you Dad, Mom, Jules, Bella, and Senior, for thinking everything I do is awesome. Thank you Marilyn Wann, Susan Stinson, Kate Harding and the gang at Shapely Prose, and the Fatosphere altogether, for stirring shit up and keeping it going. Thank you to Amy Scholder and everyone at the Feminist Press for believing in what I do. And thank you to every single person who follows me on Twitter, reads my blog, and chases my name around various media to read whatever I'm working on. Seriously. I learned pretty much everything I know from talking with you.